the 8-week
blood sugar diet
cookbook

From the team behind *The 8-Week Blood Sugar Diet Cookbook*

The 8-Week Blood Sugar Diet (Dr. Michael Mosley)

The FastLife (Dr. Michael Mosley with Mimi Spencer and Peta Bee)

The FastBeach Diet (Mimi Spencer, foreword by Dr. Michael Mosley)

FastExercise (Dr. Michael Mosley with Peta Bee)

The FastDiet Cookbook (Dr. Sarah Schenker with Mimi Spencer, foreword by Dr. Michael Mosley)

The FastDiet (Dr. Michael Mosley with Mimi Spencer)

the 8-week blood sugar diet cookbook

DR. CLARE BAILEY WITH
Dr. Sarah Schenker

PHOTOGRAPHY BY JOE SARAH

ATRIA PAPERBACK
NEW YORK   LONDON   TORONTO   SYDNEY   NEW DELHI

Disclaimer: This publication contains the opinions and ideas of its authors. It is intended to provide helpful and informative material on the subjects addressed in the publication. It is not intended as and should not be relied upon as medical advice. It is sold with the understanding that the authors and publisher are not engaged in rendering medical, health, or any other kind of personal or professional services in the book. The reader should consult his or her medical, health, or other competent professional before adopting any of the suggestions in this book or drawing inferences from it. The authors and publisher specifically disclaim all responsibility for any liability, loss, or risk, personal or otherwise, which is incurred as a consequence, directly or indirectly, of the use and applications of any of the contents of this book. If you have underlying health problems, or have any doubts about the information contained in this book, you should contact a qualified medical, dietary, or other appropriate professional.

ATRIA PAPERBACK
An Imprint of Simon & Schuster, Inc.
1230 Avenue of the Americas
New York, NY 10020

Copyright © 2016 by Parenting Matters Ltd.

Originally published in Great Britain in 2016 by Short Books as *The 8-Week Blood Sugar Diet Recipe Book*
Published by arrangement with Short Books Limited

All rights reserved, including the right to reproduce this book or portions thereof in any form whatsoever. For information, address Atria Books Subsidiary Rights Department, 1230 Avenue of the Americas, New York, NY 10020.

First Atria Paperback edition December 2016

ATRIA PAPERBACK and colophon are trademarks of Simon & Schuster, Inc.

For information about special discounts for bulk purchases, please contact Simon & Schuster Special Sales at 1-866-506-1949 or business@simonandschuster.com.

The Simon & Schuster Speakers Bureau can bring authors to your live event. For more information or to book an event, contact the Simon & Schuster Speakers Bureau at 1-866-248-3049 or visit our website at www.simonspeakers.com.

Manufactured in the United States of America

10 9 8 7 6 5 4 3 2 1

Library of Congress Cataloging-in-Publication Data
Names: Bailey, Clare, author. | Schenker, Sarah, author.
Title: The 8-week blood sugar diet cookbook / Dr. Clare Bailey with Dr. Sarah
  Schenker.
Other titles: 8-Week blood sugar diet recipe book | Eight-week blood sugar
  diet cookbook
Description: New York : Atria Paperbacks, 2016. | Revision of: 8-Week blood
  sugar diet recipe book.
Identifiers: LCCN 2016038197 (print) | LCCN 2016039705 (ebook) |
Subjects: LCSH: Reducing diets—Recipes. | Sugar-free diet—Recipes. |
  Diabetes—Diet therapy—Recipes. | BISAC: COOKING / Health & Healing /
  Weight Control. | HEALTH & FITNESS / Diets. | HEALTH & FITNESS / Weight
  Loss. | LCGFT: Cookbooks.
Classification: LCC RM222.2 .B342 2016 (print) | LCC RM222.2 (ebook) | DDC
  641.5/63837—dc23
LC record available at https://lccn.loc.gov/2016038197

ISBN 978-1-5011-6053-0
ISBN 978-1-5011-6055-4 (ebook)

Contents

Foreword by Dr. Michael Mosley

On my first day at medical school I sat nervously with a hundred other students in a huge lecture hall while the dean gave his usual introductory talk. It was a long time ago but I can remember two things he said. Firstly, based on previous experience, he predicted that four of us in the room would marry. He was right: I met my wife that day (more about her later). The other memorable thing he said was that, while we would learn an enormous amount during our medical training, in time much of it would become out of date. Which is why it is so important for doctors (and the rest of us) to try and keep up with the latest science.

I was mindful of this when, in 2012, I went to see my GP with a minor complaint, had a routine blood test, and discovered that I was a type 2 diabetic. I was told that I should start on medication. But I wasn't convinced that my only option was to spend a lifetime on drugs. So I started researching alternative approaches.

I came across something called "intermittent fasting" and, the more I dug, the more interesting it looked. I finally decided to make a documentary about intermittent fasting for the BBC science series, *Horizon*, with myself as the subject.

In the course of making the documentary I put myself on what I called a "5:2 diet," whereby you eat normally five days a week and cut your calories down to around 600 calories for two days. On this diet I lost about 20 pounds in 12 weeks and my blood sugar levels went back to normal. I later cowrote a book, *the FastDiet*, which became an international bestseller.

That book was not, however, aimed at diabetics and I wondered at the time why losing the weight had produced such a dramatic impact on my blood sugar levels. Then, in 2015, I met up with Dr. Roy Taylor of Newcastle University, who is one of Europe's leading diabetes experts.

It's been known for some time that too much fat around your middle (so-called visceral fat) greatly increases your risk of diabetes, heart disease, and high blood pressure. Our rapidly expanding waists have been a major driver behind the huge rise in rates of type 2 diabetes in recent times. Ideally, your waist (measured around your belly button) should be less than half your height. In other words, if you are 5 feet 9 inches tall, your waist should be less than 35 inches.

Visceral fat is particularly bad for you because it clogs up your liver and your pancreas (the organ that produces the hormone insulin, which regulates blood sugar levels). Once this happens you are on the path to becoming a diabetic.

The good news, however, is that this is not inevitable. You can do something to both prevent and reverse type 2 diabetes.

Dr. Taylor told me he and his team had shown that, if you can reduce your body weight by 10 to 15 percent, this shrinks the visceral fat, unclogs your liver and pancreas and, in the majority of diabetic patients, enables them to come off their medication.

Meanwhile, if you are a prediabetic (i.e., you have raised blood sugars but are not yet in the diabetic range) then a 10 percent reduction in body weight will cut your chance of becoming diabetic by an amazing 90 percent!

Dr. Taylor also surprised me by saying that one of the most effective ways to lose weight and keep it off is through a rapid weight-loss diet. I'd always believed that it's better to lose weight slowly and steadily, but this isn't what the latest science shows.

In clinical trials, Dr. Taylor's team has shown that going on a program of 800 calories a day for 8 weeks produces average weight loss of 30 pounds and reversal of type 2 diabetes in the majority of patients.

His work formed the basis of my most recent book, *The 8-Week Blood Sugar Diet*, and is a founding principle of this companion recipe book.

Although it sounds challenging, most people who have tried the 8-Week Blood Sugar Diet have found it easier than conventional dieting and much more rewarding. Carole, for example, wrote to me to say, *"Having followed the regime in your book I have lost 35 pounds and I no longer have diabetes. I have gone from dress size 14/16 to 10/12. My husband has lost over 44 pounds. It has been life-changing and now that we are eating differently I think my taste buds have changed. I find so much more flavor in food."*

As Carole hints, it isn't just about cutting your calories, it is also about changing what you eat. I keep my weight off and my blood sugar levels down by minimizing sugary and starchy carbs and instead eating a low-carb, Mediterranean-style diet. This is one which is rich in vegetables, fruit, fish, meat, nuts, and olive oil—and which allows the occasional glass of wine and chocolate, just not the bread, pasta, and potatoes. It's the approach that informs the recipes in this book, which were created by Dr. Clare Bailey and Dr. Sarah Schenker.

Sarah is a registered dietitian and nutritionist. We've worked together on a number of previous books. I rate her highly.

I am also a big fan of Dr. Clare Bailey, a general practitioner who just happens to be my wife. As I mentioned earlier we met at medical school, and ever since I've known her she has been passionate about food. She is one of those annoying people who stays slim, seemingly without effort. Her secret is that she rarely snacks and she has always enjoyed a Mediterranean style of eating.

She loves trying different ingredients, different combinations, but she also wanted to produce recipes that are not too complicated or expensive. As a family we have greatly enjoyed testing and tasting the recipes in this book.

Clare's motivation for writing it comes from the fact that as a doctor she has seen so many of her patients do well using the 8-Week Blood Sugar Diet approach. This includes Cassie, an insulin-dependent diabetic who lost 66 pounds on the diet and who managed to not only come off all medication but also improve her PCOS (polycystic ovary syndrome). After several years of trying, Cassie recently got pregnant and gave birth to twins.

The joy of this diet is that it is extremely flexible. We are all different and have different needs. So, though many people will opt for the intensive 800-calorie approach to achieve the greatest impact and quickest result, you can go more gently. I know people who have started off consuming 800 calories every day, then moved to a slightly more relaxed regime of 800 calories five days a week. Some do the diet two days a week; others have simply changed to the low-blood-sugar way of eating, watching their carb intake, reducing portion sizes but not constantly counting calories. As Lisa recently wrote, *"If you can't cope with 800 I would just up it a little. My mum has lost 8 pounds and as she is inactive that's brilliant. Her blood sugar is more stable than ever and she's looking great. Give it a go, it could change your life!"*

So, do you want to lose weight, improve your health, and get your blood sugars under control? Do you want to do this while eating tasty, filling food? If so, you are in the right place. To eat and to live. That is what this book is all about.

Introduction by Dr. Clare Bailey

"Jack Sprat could eat no fat. His wife could eat no lean.

And so between them both, you see, they licked the platter clean."

Michael and I used to be like Jack Sprat and his wife. Twenty years ago, worried about his health, Michael followed standard dietary advice and cut down on fat. I, however, continued to eat what I liked, a diet which included its fair share of fats. Over the next decade he expanded around the middle and developed type 2 diabetes. And I, conversely, seemed to maintain a steady weight. Perhaps the dietary advice we'd been given was wrong?

Well, yes, as it turned out. Cutting out fat, as we now know, both deprives us of a key source of nutrients and tends to lead to an increase in the consumption of other, more pernicious things, like refined carbohydrates. This is just one of the dietary misconceptions that Michael has highlighted in the course of his research into fasting and weight loss. Most recently, in his book *The 8-Week Blood Sugar Diet* he has drawn on new evidence to transform the way we think about food.

Before Michael started his research, as a GP I would typically have told a newly diagnosed type 2 diabetic that they should go on a low-fat diet, cut down on sugar, and try to lose some weight. Unfortunately, because this rarely worked, the next step was usually medication.

These days my approach is very different. When I see someone with raised blood sugars I start by explaining that much of the dietary advice we've been giving them for the last few decades has been unhelpful and that there's a lot of science which supports a new approach, involving rapid weight loss as a means of reducing and controlling blood sugar levels. I tell them that once they move away from basing their diet on starchy carbohydrates and sugars they will find that they no longer feel hungry all the time; that their body's natural feedback mechanisms will kick back into action to switch off hunger signals and tell them when they are full.

At this point they normally look hugely relieved. Most, though not all, are then keen to give it a go and those who persist with the Blood Sugar Diet typically see impressive reductions in blood sugar levels within a matter of weeks. They also see significant weight loss and a reduction in waist circumference, often around 2 to 4 inches.

For any of you who have not read Michael's book, *The 8-Week Blood Sugar Diet* sets out a bold and radical program that involves you sticking to around 800 calories a day for up to 8 weeks. This intensive approach is the fastest way to see change, and the recipes in this book have been designed with that goal in mind. Your calorie intake can be averaged out over the week so it's fine to go up to 900 on some days and down to 700 on others. It does not have to be absolutely exact. All the calorie counts in the recipes here are calculated for a single portion, and, in the spirit of pragmatism, we have rounded them to the nearest 10.

As Michael pointed out in his foreword, the recipes are all based on a Mediterranean style of eating because this has the most rigorous scientific backing when it comes to losing weight and improving blood sugar levels. The other really important thing is that numerous studies have shown that people find this approach satisfying and sustainable, and so you are far more likely to stick to it than to a conventional low-fat diet.

Over the past few years, we have made a conscious effort at home to shift towards a lower-carbohydrate, higher-fat diet, one rich in olive oil, fish, nuts, fruit, and vegetables, as well as lots of delicious things that down the years we have been told to avoid, such as full-fat yogurt and eggs. I love this sort of food and I have thoroughly enjoyed putting the theory behind the diet into practice—developing the recipes for this book.

I hope you will enjoy them, too. I have been much cheered by the feedback from my patients, many of whom say that it's the first diet they've felt they can stick to.

No one diet is going to suit everyone. So if you find that 800 calories a day, every day, is too tough to sustain, then, as Michael recommends, you could try the gentler 5:2 approach in which you eat 800 calories two days a week.

On the other five days you should follow a Mediterranean-style way of eating, but without strictly counting calories. This can be done using the recipes in this book, often by simply doubling portion sizes and adding extras to some of your meals such as an additional salad or portion of vegetables or a couple of tablespoons of lentils, beans, bulgur wheat, or quinoa. You might add more nuts, seeds, whole grains, and the occasional piece of whole grain bread. You won't reach your goals quite as fast with this approach, but it is still effective.

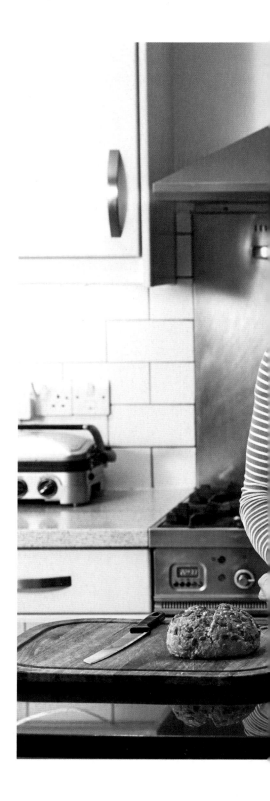

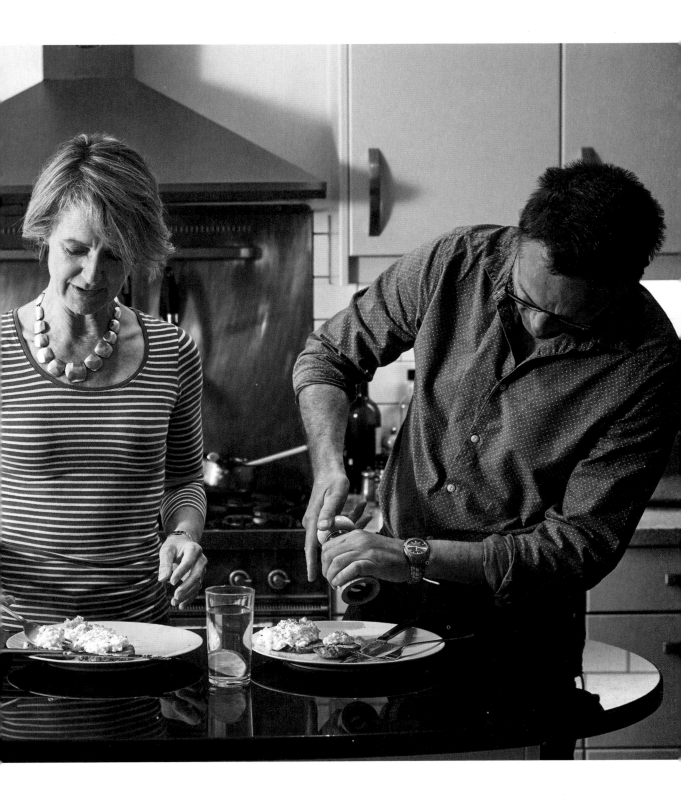

About the 8-Week Blood Sugar Diet

The 8-Week Blood Sugar Diet is based on a Mediterranean style of eating—one which is low in starchy, easily digestible carbs, but packed full of disease-fighting vitamins and flavonoids. Numerous trials have shown that not only do people get multiple health benefits from this diet, but they are also good at sticking to it (unlike those who go on a low-fat diet) because they find it easy and enjoyable. Although it is derived from the eating habits of people living in Mediterranean countries, you can apply the principles of Med-style eating to a wide range of cuisines, from Chinese or Indian through to Mexican or Scandinavian, as we have done in this book.

7 principles for low-carb Mediterranean-style eating

1. **Minimize or avoid the "white stuff."** The main culprits are bread, pasta, potatoes, processed cereals, and rice—all refined and starchy carbohydrates which rapidly turn into sugars in the blood. Switch instead to quinoa, whole grains, beans, and lentils as these are good and filling, too. Avoid just going brown: brown rice is OK, but some whole wheat breads contain added sugar, and the extra fiber added usually only has a small impact on reducing the carbohydrate load.

2. **Cut right down on sugar, sugary treats, drinks, and desserts.** We offer plenty of recipes for healthy alternatives. The aim is to wean yourself off sugar.

3. **Eat more vegetables.** In fact, eat a rainbow, from purple beets through red and yellow peppers to dark leafy greens . . . Non-starchy vegetables are also a great way to top up on all those vital phytonutrients. We include lots of tips and simple recipes to make your vegetables irresistibly

delicious in the hope that this will encourage even the more reluctant vegetable eaters to increase their intake so that vegetables makes up half of every plate.

4. **Include some fruit, but ideally not more than 1 to 2 portions daily.** Go for berries, apples, and pears—unpeeled, as this is where most of the nutrients are. And avoid or minimize your intake of high-sugar "tropical" fruits such as mango, pineapple, melon, and bananas.

5. **Include plenty of high-quality protein (at least 1½ to 2 ounces per day).** The body doesn't store protein, so you need to maintain an adequate level in your diet to avoid muscle loss. It also helps to reduce appetite. Processed meats (e.g., bacon, salami, sausages) should be eaten in moderation. High-quality proteins include meat, oily fish, eggs, seafood, tofu, soy, and, to a lesser extent nuts, chickpeas, quinoa, lentils.

6. **Enjoy your dairy products and eat more healthy fats and oils.** Until recently full-fat dairy products were shunned because of a misguided fear that they are bad for you. In 2014 a systematic review by the British Heart Foundation* which looked at the results of nearly 80 studies involving more than half a million people found no evidence that eating saturated fats leads to a greater risk of heart disease. In fact, they found that people with higher levels in their blood of a particular saturated fat called margaric acid (the sort you get in milk and dairy products) had a lower risk of heart disease. These days I encourage people to consume more fats such as olive oil, yogurt, cheese, nuts, shrimp, avocados, and coconut milk. They make food taste better. They are an excellent source of slow-burn energy. And, although ounce for ounce they are higher in calories than carbs, they keep you full for longer. Adding fat to starchy food (butter to potatoes, for example), will actually slow the rate at which the starch is broken down into sugars and absorbed. Eating healthy oils also improves the absorption of the essential fat-soluble vitamins (A, D, E, and K).

7. **Bring on the vinegar!** Vinegar has been found to help reduce weight and visceral (abdominal) fat, improve lipids and insulin sensitivity, so not surprisingly it features in a number of recipes in this book. In a recent study,** scientists found that adding 2 teaspoons of vinegar to a meal cut the post-meal blood sugar spike by 20%, while subjects in another study,*** who were asked to consume a tablespoon of vinegar a day for 12 weeks, lost about 4 ounces more than those taking a placebo drink. Vinegar has been shown to suppress appetite and it also delays the breakdown of food into sugars in your gut.

---

* Association of dietary, circulating and supplement fatty acids with coronary risk http://annals. org/article.aspx?articleid=1846638)

** http://www.ncbi.nlm.nih.gov/pubmed/20068289

*** http://www.ncbi.nlm.nih.gov/pubmed/19661687

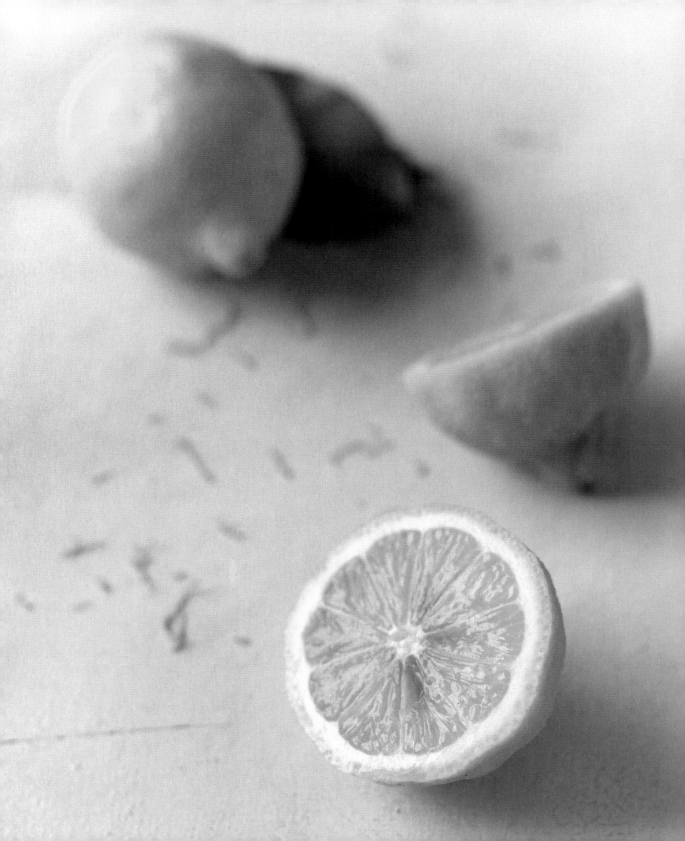

Some common questions

What are GI and GL?

Glycemic Index (GI) is a measure of the rate at which the food you eat causes your blood sugars to rise. Low-GI foods cause blood sugar levels to rise more slowly than high-GI foods, and this helps you to feel fuller for longer. Refined and starchy carbohydrates normally have a high GI; this means they cause a spike in blood sugar levels, which then crash, leaving you feeling hungry again and so encouraging you to eat more.

The size of the spike in blood sugars is not just a result of the type of food you eat, but the amount—which is measured in Glycemic Load (GL). Eating a big bowl of pasta is going to produce a larger, more sustained spike than eating a small bowl. For more information, go to: http://www.glycemicindex.com/.

As a rule of thumb, be wary of carbs with a GI over 50, or a GL over 20, such as pasta, bread, and processed cereals. Switching to lower GL versions of these staples can produce impressive improvements in blood sugar control. You should also be aware that GI and GL only relate to carbs. You won't find foods rich in protein or fat (such as chicken or butter) listed in the database above as they don't significantly affect blood sugar levels.

Can I use sweeteners?

Ideally not. We have tried to avoid use of sweeteners of any kind in our recipes, because they tend to perpetuate hunger signals and sugar cravings. Part of the aim is to help people lose their sweet tooth. So for the occasional sweet treat we aim to use sugar from fruit such as dates or include a small amount of maple syrup.

Which fats should I cook with?

Olive oil and rapeseed oil are rich in "monounsaturated fats," which are also found in avocados, olives, almonds, and hazelnuts. Monounsaturated fats are not only good for you when they are cold, they are also better at resisting damage caused by heating than the polyunsaturated fats found in sunflower and other vegetable oils. When fats and oils are heated to "smoke point" (when frying or baking) they undergo oxidation: they react with oxygen in the air to form aldehydes and lipid peroxides. Consuming or inhaling these, even in small amounts, has been linked to increased risk of cancer and heart disease. We have chosen olive, rapeseed, and coconut oils for this book as they release less of these nasty aldehydes.

We like coconut oil in particular because of its flavor, but also because there's evidence it can be helpful in reducing central obesity (i.e., visceral fat). In one study,* 40 female volunteers were randomly allocated to either 1 ounce (2 tablespoons) of coconut oil or soybean oil per day for 12 weeks. Unlike those consuming soybean oil, the women consuming coconut oil saw significant reductions in waist size and improvements in their cholesterol profile. For drizzling on salads and over vegetables, you might prefer the stronger, slightly nutty flavor of extra-virgin olive oil. Continue to avoid foods containing trans fats (present in many processed foods and some margarines).

Can I snack?

We recommend you keep snacking to a minimum. In the time between meals your body has a chance to go into fat-burning and repair mode. That said, we understand many people starting this diet have had fairly haphazard eating patterns as a result of busy lives and may have ended up relying on starchy meals and snacks. To counter this, we include lots of options for practical and healthy light meals or snacks to keep the wolf from the door.

How can I stay motivated?

If you are clear about why you are doing this diet, and what you want to get out of it, you will find sticking to it much easier. Consider your GOAL:

Get. What do you want to get out of it? What target do you want to get to? Is your main aim to reach a specific weight? If so, write it down. Is it to improve raised blood sugars? What level are you aiming for? To reverse diabetes? To avoid starting extra medication or starting insulin? And what is motivating you to get there?

Opportunities. What resources or opportunities do you have around you? Family? Friends? Professionals? Diet buddy? You could join the community at www.thebloodsugardiet.com

Approach. How will you approach this? What do you need to do before you start? Set up a diet diary first?

Look for successes. Little by little, you should find this new approach will improve your life in all sorts of unforeseen ways. Notice the positive changes along the way and celebrate them—whether it is improved blood sugars, blood pressure or blood lipids, losing weight, or simply having more energy and feeling better. Enjoy the change.

---

* http://www.ncbi.nlm.nih.gov/pubmed/19437058

Who should *not* follow a low-calorie diet?

You should avoid a low-calorie/fasting diet if you are: underweight and/or have a history of an eating disorder, are under 18 years of age, are pregnant or breastfeeding, have a significant psychiatric disorder, or are recovering from surgery. It is unwise to diet if you are unwell, frail or have a fever, or if you are under active investigation or treatment, or have a significant medical condition. You should consult your doctor before starting any diet, particularly if you are on certain medications such as warfarin, insulin or drugs for diabetes or blood pressure. Likewise if you are a type 1 diabetic.

It can be helpful to confirm with your doctor that you really are a type 2 diabetic as there are other rarer forms of diabetes that will not respond in the same way to weight loss. A gentler approach may be more suitable—simply following a low-carb, Med-style approach, in which you watch your portions but don't count the calories. You can use these recipes as a guide to do that, doubling quantities, and adding extra vegetables and non-starchy foods. Although it takes longer, many people get on well with this approach.

How do I work with my health professionals?

Many doctors and health professionals are already enthusiastically on board and supporting patients doing the Blood Sugar Diet, with considerable success. Some are even doing it themselves. However, there are also health professionals who are understandably cautious about supporting new diets with which they are unfamiliar.

It may help to print the following document from Dr. Roy Taylor who has helped many patients to successfully reverse their diabetes on an 800-calorie a day diet. He is a world-renowned diabetologist and has produced lots of research demonstrating the health benefits of the diet. Go to http://www.ncl .ac.uk/magres/research/diabetes/documents/Informationfordoctors_revised_ April14.pdf.

Either way, before you start, if you have not had your blood tested for diabetes and raised blood lipids, or your blood pressure, weight, and waist measured recently, it would be worth doing so. There are some helpful tests for assessing your diabetes risk on our website thebloodsugardiet.com.

Calorie counts and nutritional information

All calorie counts and nutritional information in these recipes are calculated per portion.

Getting started

First things first—a bit of kitchen hygiene. This doesn't mean getting the bleach out. It means removing those temptations hidden in the corners of your kitchen drawers—chocolate, Nutella . . . whatever it is that might test your resolve.

Blood Sugar Diet pantry essentials

If you do quite a bit of cooking, you probably already have a lot of the things on the list below. However, if you are relatively new to cooking or you are going to radically change your diet and way of eating with this book, you may find it useful to go through your kitchen cupboards and then stock up at the local supermarket. You certainly don't need to buy everything on the list. But you are more likely to cook something if you have most of what you need in store.

Some of these ingredients may look unfamiliar and some frighteningly wholesome, but bear with us and try them if you can, as variety is hugely important to your diet and we are hoping to introduce you to an enjoyable and healthier way of eating. Some of the ingredients were new to us, too. We are still having fun working out interesting and tasty things to make with chia seeds. (We have marked with asterixes the items that we use a lot.)

Spices

cardamom pods*
cayenne pepper
Chinese 5-spice
cinnamon (ground or sticks)
cumin (ground & seeds)*
curry powder (or paste)
garam masala
nutmeg
paprika*
piri piri flavoring
red pepper flakes*
sea/table salt*
spice mix
turmeric (ground)

Herbs

bay leaves (fresh or dried)
coriander (ground)
oregano*
tarragon
thyme*

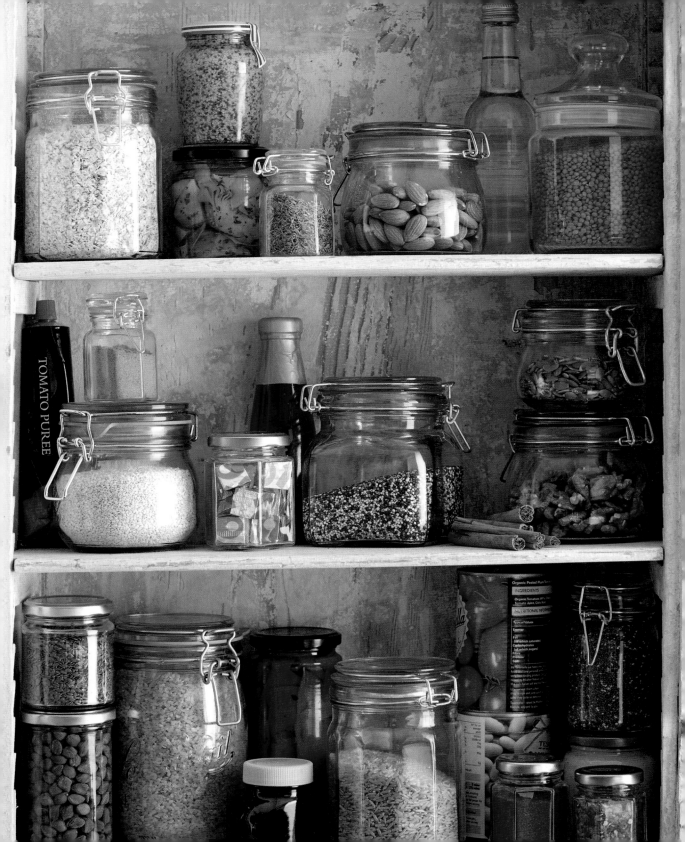

Grains, beans, and legumes

baked beans (low-sugar)
black beans (canned)
brown rice*
bulgur wheat*
butter beans (canned or dried)
cannellini beans (canned or dried)*
chickpeas (canned or dried)*
cranberry beans (canned)*
kidney beans (canned)*
lentils: black, red or green (canned, dried,
  or in packets)
oats (whole and rolled)*
quinoa*

Nuts and seeds

almonds (whole, flaked and/or ground)*
Brazil nuts
cashew nuts*
chia seeds*
flaxseeds
hazelnuts
pecans
pine nuts*
pumpkin seeds
sesame seeds
walnuts

Oils and vinegars

balsamic vinegar*
cider vinegar*
coconut oil*
extra-virgin olive oil*
olive oil*
rapeseed oil
sesame oil

Flours and baking

almond flour
baking powder*
cocoa powder (unsweetened)
cornstarch
gram flour
ground almonds*
whole wheat flour
spelt*
rye

Mustards, sauces, and pastes

basil pesto
chili paste
chutney or pickle
coconut cream
coconut milk (full-fat)*
harissa paste
hoisin sauce
honey
ginger paste
ginger (in syrup)
maple syrup
mayonnaise (full-fat)
mirin (Japanese rice wine)
miso paste
mustard (Dijon and grainy)*
soy sauce (preferably low-salt)*
stock cubes (chicken and vegetable)*
sweet chili sauce
Tabasco
Thai fish sauce*
tomato sauce*
Worcestershire sauce

Canned fish

anchovies*
sardines*
tuna*

Vegetables and fruit in cans or jars

artichoke hearts
bean sprouts
black or green olives*
capers
grapefruit
lychees
roasted red peppers
sushi pickled ginger (optional)
tomatoes*

Jams and spreads

cashew or almond nut butter

In the freezer

chicken breasts (individually wrapped)
cooked brown rice, quinoa, bulgur
  wheat (in portions)
edamame beans
fish (salmon fillet, cod, or other white fish)
fruits (berries, rhubarb, plums)
peas*
shrimp*
spinach*

Dried fruit

apricots
dates*
raisins

In the fridge

berries (raspberries, blueberries, strawberries*)
cheese (Parmesan, sharp Cheddar, feta,
  halloumi)
chilies*
crème fraîche
free-range eggs
fresh ginger*
full-fat Greek yogurt
garlic*
lemons and limes
non-starchy vegetables (bell peppers, broccoli,
  cauliflower, cherry tomatoes, cucumber,
  greens, lettuce, radishes, zucchini)

Useful equipment

nonstick saucepans
nonstick frying pan and wok
nonstick omelet pan
cast-iron casserole dish suitable for stovetops
  as well as ovens
ramekins for baking small portions
short wooden skewers (for kebabs)
potato masher
lemon squeezer
spiralizer (see page 107)
large and small measuring cups
food processor or immersion blender
blender

12 TIPS for 800-cal fasting days

1. Plan in advance and aim for variety to maintain interest and nutritional balance. Many people have meals planned, or even ready the day before, so they don't give into temptation. We suggest ideas for quick and easy dishes to assemble the night before so you can dash out in the morning with a healthy breakfast on board, as well as tips for preparing something that you can have ready and waiting for you when you get home from work.

   The first 2 weeks might be tough, but most people find their body gets used to it. As their stomach shrinks and their insulin resistance improves, most people find their constant cravings settle and they don't want so much to eat. In fact, the majority of people say that they feel hugely better and have more energy.

2. Increase water intake to reduce the side effects of calorie cutting, such as tiredness, lightheadedness, and headaches (these are often related to dehydration and sometimes insufficient salt intake), hunger (this comes in waves and passes so try to "surf the wave") and feeling colder. Aim for 2 to 3 quarts a day. You can also add a bit more salt to food.

3. Drink soup as it's surprisingly satiating as well as cheap and practical. You can take it to work for lunch and keep portions in the freezer.

4. Use low-carb alternatives for potatoes, pasta, and rice. We have included all sorts of tips and tricks to help you with this. Try grated cauliflower instead of rice, spiralized vegetables or finely sliced cabbage instead of pasta or noodles.

5. Avoid sugar and sweet syrups wherever possible, even if they are "natural" sugars. Where a savory dish needs a touch of sweetness use whole fruit if you can; its impact is reduced when it is eaten with fats and fiber, which slows its absorption.

6. Drink hot drinks to suppress your appetite: teas, coffee, miso soup, etc.

7. Beware hidden calories in drinks. Alcohol is surprisingly high-calorie so avoid it if possible during the diet. Other unexpected liquid calories include fruit juice, smoothies, and cordials.

8. Avoid "diet" products as they often contain sugar and/or sweeteners to make them more palatable. And they don't reduce sweet cravings.

9. Build in strong flavors with the likes of lemon, pepper, lime, red pepper flakes, garlic, gherkins, mustard, and herbs. It is a great way of making food more satisfying.

10. Use a nutritional counter such as My Fitness Pal to measure and track your meals, especially if you are not always following the menu planner in this book, to ensure that you get a healthy nutritional balance in your diet.

11. Take multivitamins at least every other day, if you can, particularly if you are doing 800 calories for more than a few weeks. The recipes have been designed to ensure that you get a balanced diet with adequate protein, fat, and nutrients but a multivitamin won't hurt.

12. Share meals with others where possible. It is important not to become isolated on any diet. Just remember to have smaller portions of the same food where you can and skip the carbs. Friends and family might benefit, too.

What do I do once I have achieved my goals?

Once you have reached your target weight and/or got your blood sugars down to healthy levels, it is vital that you do not slip back into a starchy or high-sugar diet as that will eventually undo all the good work. So for maintenance we recommend the Blood Sugar Diet Way of Life.*

The recipes in this book provide an excellent basis for healthy eating and keeping weight and blood sugar down indefinitely. When you are no longer counting the calories, use the recipes as a guide, sticking to the principles of the Mediterranean way of eating, and simply increasing the quantities to roughly double, adding more non-starchy vegetables and including more whole grain foods. Some people, when they come off the intensive diet, continue to do an 800-calorie day once or even twice a week to keep their weight and blood sugars on track.

What we hope, above all, is that you have absorbed enough about the core principles of healthy eating from this book to be able to build them into a flexible and sustainable way of life that suits you personally. That is when dieting is successful.

* For more advice and support we recommend you join the active and well-informed community at thebloodsugardiet.com

Breakfast and Brunch

Breakfast tends to be the most underrated meal of the day, often eaten on your feet, and made up of instant cereals or a piece of toast and jam—neither of which will keep you going. The starchy carbs are burned quickly and send your blood sugars soaring, only to crash a few hours later to leave you bewilderingly hungry and craving a midday snack.

We predict a revolution in breakfast-eating habits over the next decade—one in which Blood Sugar dieters will be ahead of the game. Prepare to banish those dreary old processed cereals for good. Start the day instead with an energy-boosting combination of protein and plants: eggs, avocados, fish, tomatoes, mushrooms, spinach . . . we guarantee you will never look back.

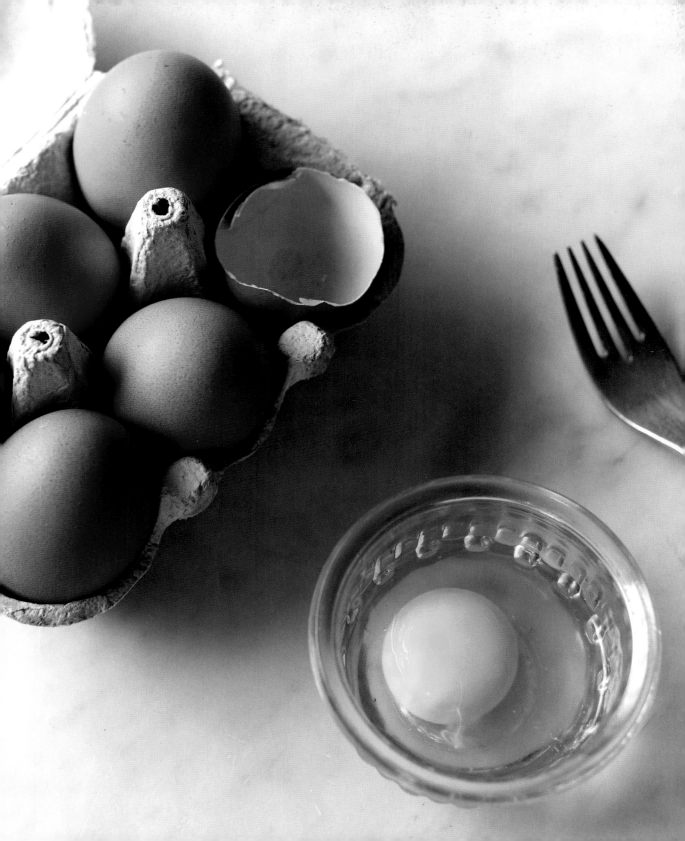

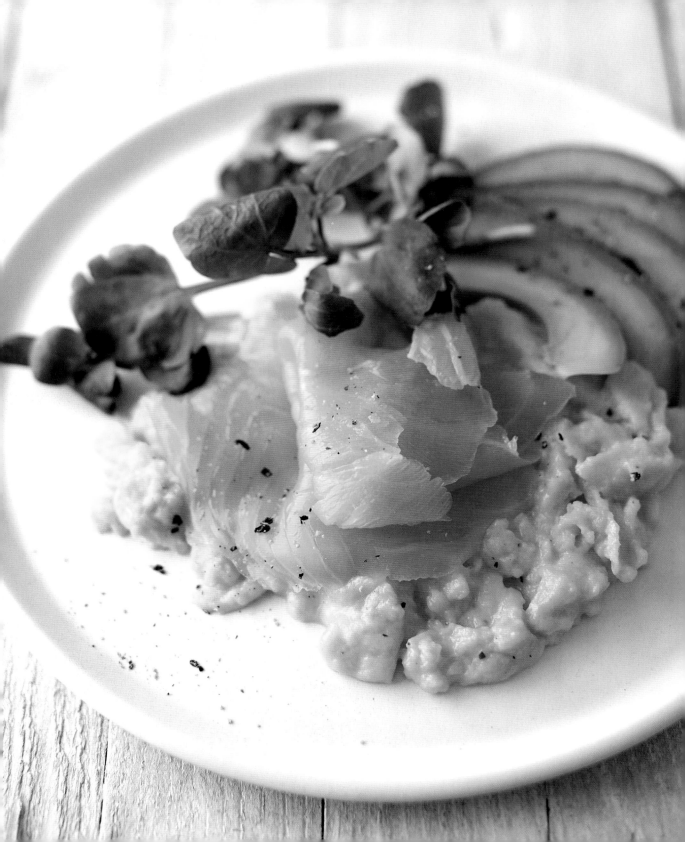

Quick, easy breakfasts

Michael's perfect scrambled eggs

Serves 1

2 eggs
Small pat of butter
(or dash of oil)

Whisk the eggs in a cup or bowl with a fork. In a small nonstick pan, heat the butter gently until it melts (don't allow it to brown), then add the eggs. Stir slowly and continuously with a wooden spoon or spatula for 1 to 2 minutes to produce a creamy consistency. Remove from the heat while it is still runny in places as it will go on cooking in the pan.

Try some of the variations below, all made with 2 eggs:

With chili: add flavor with a scattering of red pepper flakes or fresh chives.

With smoked salmon: (adds 90 calories) this is Michael's routine breakfast. Scramble 2 eggs, and serve with 2 oz chopped smoked salmon and freshly ground black pepper. You can also add ¼ medium avocado, sliced (adds 60 calories).

With fried mushrooms: (adds 20 calories) mushrooms are low in carbs, high in protein and fiber and amazingly filling given their low calorie count. They also contain high levels of vitamin D. Fry 3 oz mushrooms in a nonstick pan with a drizzle of oil until golden brown (4 to 5 minutes). Meanwhile, prepare the scrambled eggs. Assemble on a plate and season with salt and black pepper.

Green eggs and ham: (adds 50 calories) this is an excellent way to use up leftover greens from the night before. Simply stir in a handful, or some fresh spinach. Serve with a couple of slices of ham, 1½ to 2 oz.

- **CALORIES** 200
- PROTEIN 13G
- FAT 17G
- FIBER 0G
- CARBS 0G

Why we love eggs

Eggs are nutrient-dense, vitamin-rich, high in protein and healthy fatty acids, naturally vacuum-wrapped, fast to cook, and incredibly flexible. They also keep you full for longer, without pushing up your blood sugars or cholesterol. Yes! Many of my patients are surprised to hear me recommending eggs, a legacy of the years in which they were unfairly blamed for raising blood cholesterol levels. Let me reassure you: eggs are fine.

Simple omelet

Delicious on its own or with tasty extras thrown in.

Serves 1

2 eggs
Small pat of butter
  (or a dash of oil)

Gently whisk the eggs with a fork in a cup or bowl. Add pepper and salt to taste. In a small nonstick frying pan, heat the butter and spread it around the pan until it bubbles, then pour in the eggs. After a few seconds lower the heat and cook it until the underside is golden brown. Fold the omelet in half and serve it while it's still a bit runny on the surface (it will go on cooking on the plate). Perfect.

- **CALORIES** 200
- PROTEIN 13G
- FAT 17G
- FIBER 0G
- CARBS 0G

Mushroom omelet

Serves 1

3 oz mushrooms, sliced
2 eggs
Small pat of butter
  (or a dash of oil)

Sauté the mushrooms in a drizzle of oil until they are golden brown (4 to 5 minutes). Gently whisk the eggs with a fork in a cup or bowl. Add salt and pepper to taste. For the omelet, heat the butter in a small nonstick frying pan, and spread it around the pan until it bubbles, then pour in the eggs. After a few seconds lower the heat, add the cooked mushrooms and cook the omelet until the underside is golden brown. Fold it in half and serve it while it is still a bit runny on the surface (it will go on cooking on the plate).

- **CALORIES** 210
- PROTEIN 14G
- FAT 17G
- FIBER 1G
- CARBS 0G

Poached eggs with spinach and pine nuts

Serves 1

1 tsp wine or cider vinegar
2 eggs
1 tsp butter
7 oz fresh spinach
¼ tsp ground nutmeg
1 tbsp grated Parmesan
1 tsp pine nuts, toasted

Bring a pan of water to a boil, add the vinegar and reduce the heat to a simmer. Crack the eggs into the water and poach them for 3 minutes. Melt the butter in a pan and add the spinach. Sprinkle on the nutmeg, a pinch of salt, and plenty of black pepper and allow the spinach to wilt over a gentle heat. Drain it in a colander and place it on a plate, topped with the eggs, a sprinkle of Parmesan, and pine nuts.

- **CALORIES** 290
- PROTEIN 17G
- FAT 24G
- FIBER 1G
- CARBS 1G

Kipper and tomatoes

Another easy, healthy default breakfast. Kippers are good value and full of wonderful fish oils. They are very practical, too, as they keep for a few days in the fridge or can be frozen. The ones in a package take 2 to 3 minutes in a microwave—about as long as it takes to make a cup of tea. For extra oomph, sprinkle them with red pepper flakes and freshly ground black pepper.

Serves 1

1 smoked kipper or mackerel fillet
Pat of butter
4 oz tomatoes

Grill or microwave the smoked fish with a pat of butter according to instructions. Serve it on a bed of tomatoes, either cold or cooked (see overnight tomatoes, page 39).

Tip: on a non-fasting day, serve it with a small piece of seeded spelt and rye toast (see bread options on pages 180–81).

- **CALORIES** 230
- PROTEIN 10G
- FAT 20G
- FIBER 1G
- CARBS 3G

Big mushrooms with feta

These are also known as Portobello mushrooms. We received an email recently from a gentleman who said he was inclined to give up on recipes with words such as falafel, frittata, harissa, Portobello, julienne strips . . . and fair enough. For this book, we have tried to keep the names of ingredients as simple and unpretentious as possible. So "Big mushrooms" it is . . . cooked with feta and olive oil. Delicious they are, too.

Serves 1

2–2½ oz fresh spinach,
  coarsely chopped
1 oz feta, crumbled
Pinch of ground nutmeg
2-3 large flat mushrooms
1 tbsp olive oil

Preheat the oven to 350°F. Wilt the spinach in a pan, drain it well and squeeze out excess water. Place it in a bowl and stir in the feta with some salt and pepper and the nutmeg.

Remove the stalks from the mushrooms, and brush the caps all over with olive oil. Place them on a baking sheet flat side down and fill them with the spinach mixture. Bake them for 15 minutes.

- **CALORIES** 130
- PROTEIN 7G
- FAT 10G
- FIBER 2G
- CARBS 2G

Avocados with prebaked tomatoes

Avocados are brimming with essential nutrients, including potassium, B vitamins, and folic acid. They also contain large amounts of the healthy monounsaturated fat, oleic acid, and have at last been acknowledged as having beneficial, health-promoting properties similar to those of olive oil.

Serves 2

7 oz tomatoes
  (about 3 medium)
½ tsp dried tarragon,
  oregano, or rosemary
2 ripe avocados
½ tsp paprika
Pinch of red pepper flakes
  (optional)

Cut the tomatoes in half, scatter with the herbs, and bake for 30 minutes (or use prebaked tomatoes, see page 39). Cut the avocados in half, scoop out the flesh and divide it between 2 plates. Then mash it coarsely, top it with the tomatoes, and serve it with the paprika, red pepper flakes, and black pepper sprinkled over the top.

- **CALORIES** 300
- PROTEIN 4G
- FAT 29G
- FIBER 7G
- CARBS 8G

Avocado and feta bash

Serves 2

1 ripe avocado
Handful of parsley
  or basil, chopped
1 tbsp olive oil
1 tbsp walnuts, toasted
  or hazelnuts for crunch
1 oz feta, crumbled
¼ tsp red pepper flakes

Cut the avocado in half and scoop out the flesh into a bowl. Mash it with the herbs, olive oil, nuts, feta, and red pepper flakes along with some seasoning. Divide the mixture between 2 plates.

Tip: if you are on a non-fasting day you could serve it on a small piece of seeded spelt and rye bread (see page 181), toasted and lightly rubbed with garlic.

- **CALORIES** 460
- PROTEIN 9G
- FAT 46G
- FIBER 5G
- CARBS 3G

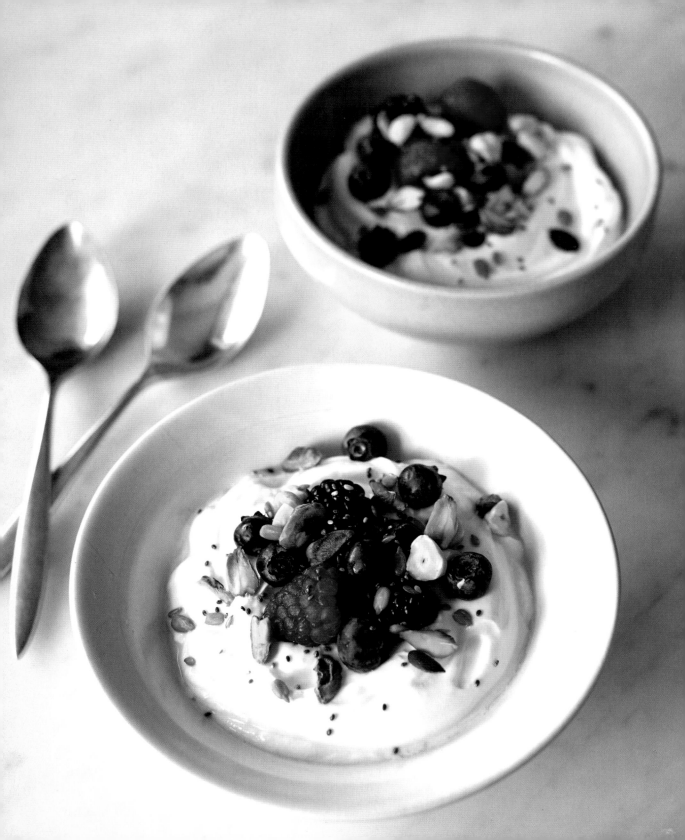

In praise of full-fat Greek yogurt

Full-fat dairy products are a staple part of the Mediterranean diet, and have now thankfully been reinstated on the official good food list, after a long time out in the cold. We generally recommend Greek-style yogurt as it has been strained to retain a higher protein content. It is satiating without significantly raising blood sugar and there is now clear evidence that a diet containing dairy products does not cause diabetes or have an undue impact on cholesterol.

Live, unsweetened yogurt will also help boost the healthy bacteria in your gut. The trouble with low-fat yogurts is that they tend to contain a lot of added sugar or sweeteners and starchy thickeners that kill these vital bacteria. So beware.

We have recently discovered full-fat coconut yogurt as a delicious nondairy alternative: it has a naturally sweet taste, is dairy-free and contains healthy fat and minimal starchy carbohydrate. It is more expensive than regular yogurt, but otherwise fits the bill.

Greek yogurt with nuts, seeds, and berries

Toasting nuts and seeds transforms their taste—the heat sets off a chemical reaction which enhances the flavor.

Serves 1

2 heaping tbsp Greek yogurt
1 tbsp toasted seeds or nuts of
your choice (sunflower seeds, pumpkin
seeds, almonds, hazelnuts, walnuts)
Small handful of berries (raspberries,
strawberries, blackberries, or
blueberries, according to
what is in season)

Assemble the yogurt, seeds, and berries and dig in.

- **CALORIES** 200
- PROTEIN 9G
- FAT 18G
- FIBER 2G
- CARBS 5G

5 ways with oatmeal

All calories are not equal, and nor are all oats. Depending on how refined or processed the oats are, there is a significant difference in impact on blood sugars. At the healthiest end of the scale is coarse oatmeal, made of relatively unrefined steel cut oats, also known as Irish oats, which retain the nutritious inner kernel, are more chewy, and require soaking and cooking for up to an hour. They have a lower GI and a slower release, keeping you fuller for longer. They contain lots of fiber, of both the soluble and insoluble kind, which contributes to keeping blood sugars down and supporting healthy gut bacteria.

Unfortunately, many people are eating "instant" oatmeal in the belief that it is good for them. Processed quick oats have less fiber and a high GI: they contain a more refined form of carbohydrate, which results in a significantly greater impact on blood sugars due to the carbohydrate being digested and released faster into the blood, making you feel hungry again, sooner.

Somewhere in between sit the jumbo oats and the slightly more processed rolled oats which are commonly used for breakfast hot cereal. We have mainly included recipes with rolled oats here, for the sake of speed and on the basis that these are certainly better for you than most breakfast cereals. But if you can, try and make sure that you have the chewy, less processed variety of oat. It takes longer to cook, but is worth it.

1. Apple and cinnamon oatmeal

Cinnamon reduces the speed at which the stomach empties and has been shown to lower blood sugar. It also has natural sweetness which helps reduce sugar intake.

Serves 1

2 heaping tbsp rolled oats
⅔ cup low-fat milk
1 apple, grated
½ tsp ground cinnamon

Put the oats and milk in a saucepan, along with the grated apple and cinnamon. Add a pinch of salt to enhance the flavors. Bring it to a boil and then simmer for about 5 minutes, stirring frequently so it doesn't stick to the bottom of the pan.

- **CALORIES** 260
- PROTEIN 9G
- FAT 9G
- FIBER 4G
- CARBS 38G

2. Extra-filling oatmeal with nut butter

Serves 1

2 heaping tbsp rolled oats
⅔ cup low-fat milk
½ tsp chia seeds

For the nut butter:
4 oz cashews (4 servings =
   ½ oz per portion)

To make the nut butter, roast the cashews on a baking sheet in the oven at 350°F for 8 to 10 minutes. Allow them to cool, then blitz them in a food processor until smooth. (The butter can be stored in a jar with a lid for up to 5 days.)

To make the oatmeal, put the oats and milk in a saucepan, along with 1 tbsp nut butter and a pinch of salt. Bring it to a boil and then simmer for about 5 minutes, stirring frequently so that it doesn't stick to the bottom of the pan. (You can also microwave it in a high-sided bowl, covered, for 3 to 4 minutes.) Scatter the chia seeds over the surface and serve.

- **CALORIES** 310
- PROTEIN 12G
- FAT 17G
- FIBER 3G
- CARBS 28G

3. Medium oatmeal

According to the latest research, coconut oil can help you lose weight and reduce "dangerous" abdominal fat. It is made up of medium-chain fatty acids that are metabolized differently from the much commoner, longer-chain fats. A study of 14 healthy men found that those who ate medium-chain fatty acids such as coconut oil at breakfast ate significantly fewer calories at lunch.*

Serves 1

1 heaping tbsp medium
   steel cut oats
⅔ cup water
⅓ cup low-fat milk
1 tsp coconut oil
½ tsp ground cinnamon
   or ginger
Pinch of salt
1 fig, chopped

Put the oats in a saucepan and soak them overnight in the water (enough to just cover them).

In the morning, add the milk, coconut oil, and cinnamon and simmer for about 5 minutes, stirring frequently. Serve it with the fig scattered on top.

- **CALORIES** 290
- PROTEIN 10G
- FAT 15G
- FIBER 3G
- CARBS 31G

---

* http://www.ncbi.nlm.nih.gov/pubmed/9701177)

4. Spicy fruit oatmeal

Serves 1

1 small apple or pear,
  skin on, cored, and diced
½ tsp spice mix
Pat of butter
1 heaping tbsp rolled oats
⅔ cup low-fat milk

Dust the apple pieces in the spice mix, fry them briefly in the butter and set them aside. Put the oats and milk in a saucepan with a pinch of salt. Bring it to a boil, then simmer for about 5 minutes, stirring frequently. Serve it with the spiced apple piled on top.

- **CALORIES** 210
- PROTEIN 9G
- FAT 5G
- FIBER 3G
- CARBS 34G

---

5. Pecan chia oatmeal with raspberries

Set yourself up for the day with this very pleasing variation on oatmeal. It has a delicate flavor which you wouldn't immediately recognize as Earl Grey and which contrasts deliciously with the berries and nuts.

Serves 2

1 Earl Grey tea bag
1 cup low-fat milk
1 tbsp chia seeds
1 heaping tbsp rolled oats
6 oz raspberries,
  strawberries, or
  blueberries
3 tbsp full-fat Greek yogurt
1 tbsp chopped pecans

Steep the tea bag in ¼ cup of boiling water for 1 minute, then stir with a teaspoon and press out excess fluid before discarding the bag.

Place the milk, chia seeds, oats, berries (reserving a few for garnish) and tea in a small saucepan and simmer for 2 to 3 minutes, stirring frequently. Let it cool slightly before transferring to a bowl.

Stir in the yogurt and cool the mixture in the fridge for 30 minutes or longer, to allow it to set a little. Top it with the remaining berries and sprinkle with the nuts.

- **CALORIES** 230
- PROTEIN 15G
- FAT 27G
- FIBER 4G
- CARBS 15G

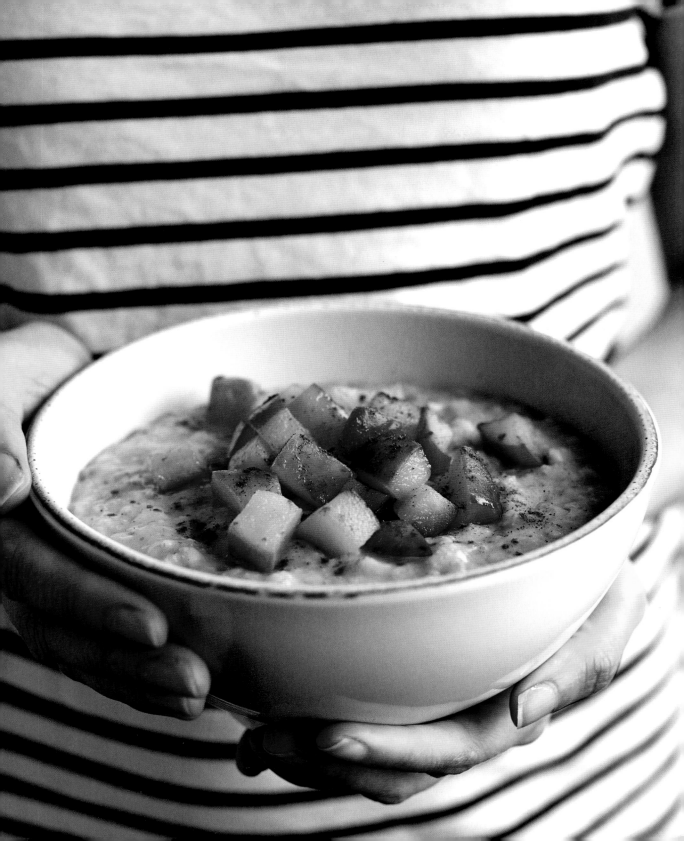

Chia breakfast bircher

Chia is amazingly high in nutrients—particularly rich in omega-3, an important fatty acid that protects the cardiovascular system and improves cholesterol. It is a relatively new discovery for us and we are enjoying its flexibility. Although it has little flavor of its own, chia seeds can be scattered over almost any food or mixed in to create a creamy texture.

Serves 2

1 tbsp chia seeds
1 heaping tbsp rolled
 oats with bran
¾ cup coconut milk
2 passion fruit
 (or a squeeze of lemon
 and zest of half a lemon)
2 ripe figs, chopped, or
 a handful of berries
1 tbsp hazelnuts, toasted
 and chopped

Combine the chia seeds, oats, and coconut milk, then divide the mixture between 2 small bowls and allow it to stand for at least 30 minutes. (It is even better prepared the night before and kept in the fridge.) Scoop out the seeds from the passion fruit and stir them into the bircher. Serve it topped with the figs and nuts.

- **CALORIES** 340
- PROTEIN 6G
- FAT 27G
- FIBER 3G
- CARBS 20G

Advance prep tips

- **Chop and put aside ingredients to add to an omelet or scrambled eggs the night before**—look out for tasty leftovers, such as a handful of meat, cheese, or cooked greens.

- **Make your oatmeal the day before** so you can simply reheat it in the microwave with an extra tablespoon of milk, depending on your preferred consistency.

- **Roast tomatoes overnight**—perfect tomatoes, ready when you wake, adapted from a neat idea by Nigella, who cooks them slowly overnight as the oven cools.

    Serves 2
    3-4 medium tomatoes, halved
    1 tsp dried thyme or tarragon
    Dash of olive oil
    Salt
    Pepper

    Preheat the oven to 400°F. Place the tomatoes cut side up on a baking dish. Scatter with the herbs, drizzle with the olive oil and season with salt and black pepper. Place the dish on the top rack of the oven and turn the oven off. By the morning, your roasted tomatoes will be ready and waiting. Serve them with kippers or half an avocado for a fantastically healthy breakfast.

- **Keep ready-toasted seeds at hand**—nuts and seeds taste sweeter toasted, so prepare a bulk batch by either dry-frying them in a pan, or browning them under the broiler or in the oven. You need to watch closely as they can burn easily. Store them in small clean jam jars with lids, ready to sprinkle on anything from yogurt or oatmeal to salads.

- **Prepare hard-boiled eggs the day before**—for an instant getaway, boil two eggs for 7 minutes, then dunk them in a bowl of cold water and pat them dry. When you're ready to eat them, simply peel them and season them with salt and pepper.

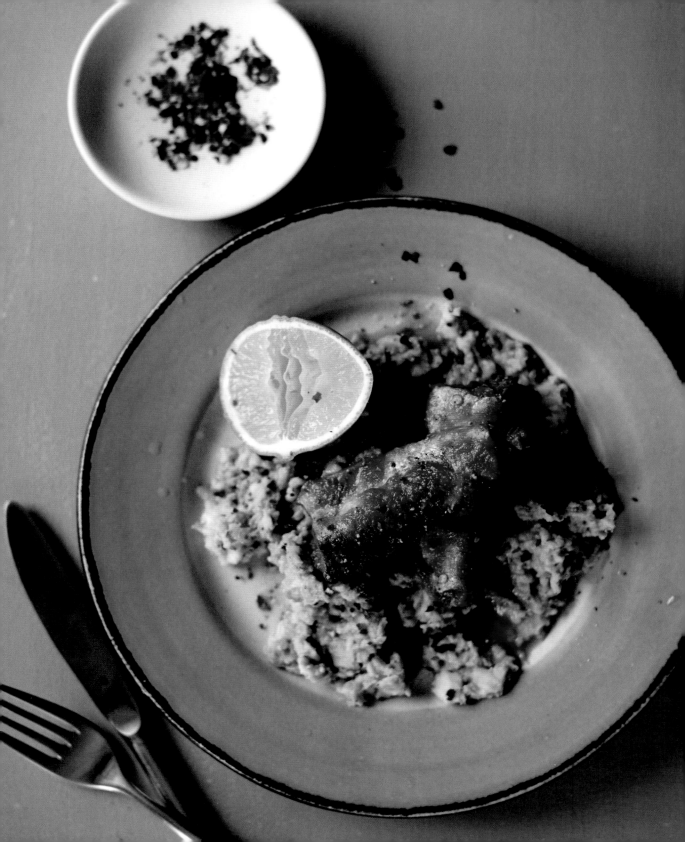

Brunch

These are more substantial dishes, perhaps best for the weekend when you get up a bit later and breakfast merges into lunch. Some take slightly longer to prepare than the quick breakfasts—but they will keep you going well into the day without a sugar spike in sight.

Sardines on avocado mash

A great combination that is incredibly filling and contains oodles of wonderful omega-3. It is also very quick to make.

Serves 1

2 oz canned sardines in
  tomato sauce
1 avocado, coarsely mashed
Squeeze of lime

Lay the sardines on top of the avocado mash, squeeze over the lime juice, and season with salt and freshly ground black pepper (red pepper flakes, too, if you like).

- **CALORIES** 370
- PROTEIN 13G
- FAT 34G
- FIBER 5G
- CARBS 4G

Ham and cheese omelet

A more substantial omelet, with a crucial extra bit of protein to keep hunger at bay.

Serves 1

2 eggs
2 oz ham, sliced
Pat of butter
 (or a dash of oil)
1 tbsp grated Cheddar

Gently whisk the eggs with a fork in a cup or bowl and add the cooked ham and salt and pepper to taste. In a small nonstick frying pan, heat the butter, and spread it around the pan until it bubbles, then pour in the mixture. After a few seconds lower the heat, sprinkle the cheese on top and cook the omelet until the underside is golden brown. Fold it in half and let it cook for about a minute more. Serve it while it's still a bit runny on the surface (it goes on cooking on the plate). Try it with a scattering of red pepper flakes to add flavor.

See pages 28 and 55 for more omelet recipes.

- **CALORIES** 340
- PROTEIN 26G
- FAT 26G
- FIBER 1G
- CARBS 0G

Simple egg muffins

Adapted from a lovely recipe on the Blood Sugar Diet website by Aliba. Easy to make with everyday ingredients and delicious hot or cold, they make an excellent portable breakfast, brunch, or lunch. Any extra muffins can be frozen.

Serves 6—makes 6 muffins in a standard muffin pan

½ cup finely chopped
 mushrooms
Small pat of butter
4 eggs
½ cup full-fat cottage
 cheese
4-5 slices bacon
1½ oz Cheddar, grated, or
 feta, crumbled
Handful of baby spinach
 leaves, shredded (or a
 handful of precooked
 greens)

Preheat the oven to 350°F. Fry the mushrooms in the butter in a nonstick pan, then set them aside. Beat the eggs with the cottage cheese and season. Cut the bacon to roughly the size needed to line the base of a 6-cup muffin pan. Add the mushrooms, cheese, and spinach to each muffin cup, pour over the egg mixture and bake for 30 to 35 minutes.

- **CALORIES** 130
- PROTEIN 11G
- FAT 10G
- FIBER 0G
- CARBS 1G

Egg baked in avocado

Serves 2

1 large avocado
Pinch of paprika
2 eggs
1 slice of smoked salmon,
  chopped
¼ red chile, seeded and
  finely chopped, or ¼ tsp
  red pepper flakes
Squeeze of lime juice

Preheat the oven to 400°F. Using a spoon, scoop out a third of the avocado flesh, leaving ¾-inch-thick walls. Place each avocado half, cut side up, in a loaf pan, to keep them upright. Sprinkle each with paprika. Crack an egg into each avocado half, and then arrange the salmon pieces evenly on top. Bake them for 10 minutes.

Meanwhile, mash the remaining avocado flesh in a small bowl and mix it with the chile, lime juice, and some black pepper to make a dip.

- **CALORIES** 230
- PROTEIN 10G
- FAT 20G
- FIBER 3G
- CARBS 1G

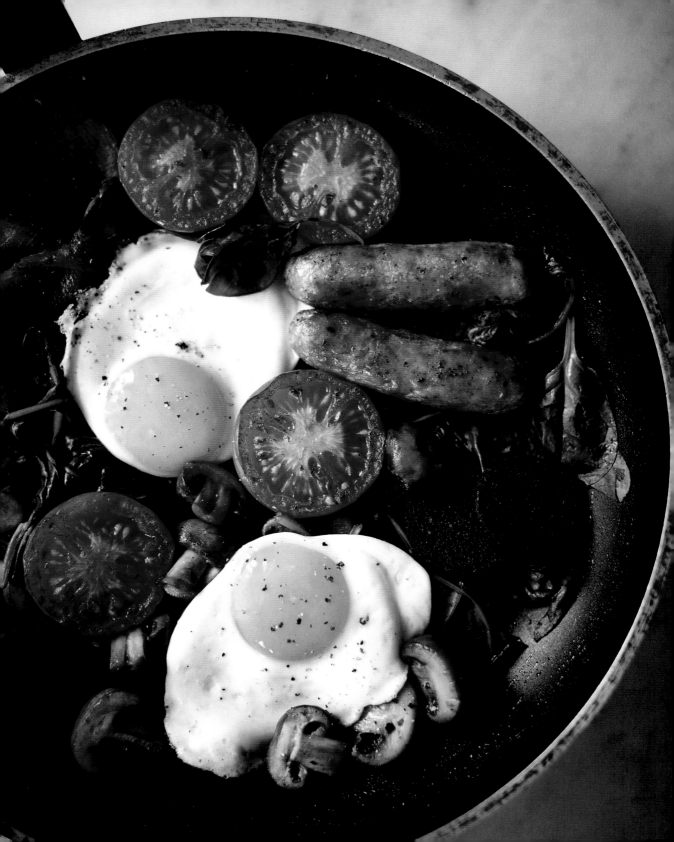

Full English breakfast

. . . just without the toast. This can be easily expanded for lots of people, and makes a great weekend treat.

Serves 2

2 tsp olive oil
2 slices free-range
  back bacon
2 good quality sausages
7 oz mushrooms, sliced
2 large slices, or 4 small
  slices black pudding or
  Andouille sausage
2 medium tomatoes,
  halved
2 eggs
8 oz spinach

Turn on the oven to 250ºF to keep things warm as you cook them. Place a large frying pan over medium to high heat, add 1 tsp olive oil and fry the bacon and sausages. Put them in an ovenproof dish in the oven. In the same oil, fry the mushrooms, and transfer them to the dish in the oven. Next fry the tomatoes for 2 to 3 minutes on each side and put them in the oven, too.

Now, add the remaining 1 tsp oil, fry the black pudding, and finally the eggs (or scramble these in a small nonstick pan if preferred). While assembling the food on 2 plates, wilt the spinach in the pan.

- **CALORIES** 330
- PROTEIN 19G
- FAT 24G
- FIBER 2G
- CARBS 9G

Quick Lunches, Smart Snacks

The people who do really well on the Blood Sugar Diet tend to be those who have identified the moments at which they are at greatest risk of breaking their good intentions. For some, this is on days when they are trying to skip lunch; for others, it is when they get back from work and need something to take the edge off their hunger. This is Michael's Achilles' heel—how to avoid going for the toast. . . .

Remember, successful dieting is less about will power than good planning. We recommend having a small portion of something tasty— a dip, nibble, healthy seed bar—ready on hand when you need it, to keep temptation at bay.

That said, we would urge you as much as possible to try and avoid snacking between meals. It's when you haven't eaten for a while that you burn fat and flush out the sugar stored in your liver and pancreas. As soon as you snack, you stop that restorative process in its tracks.

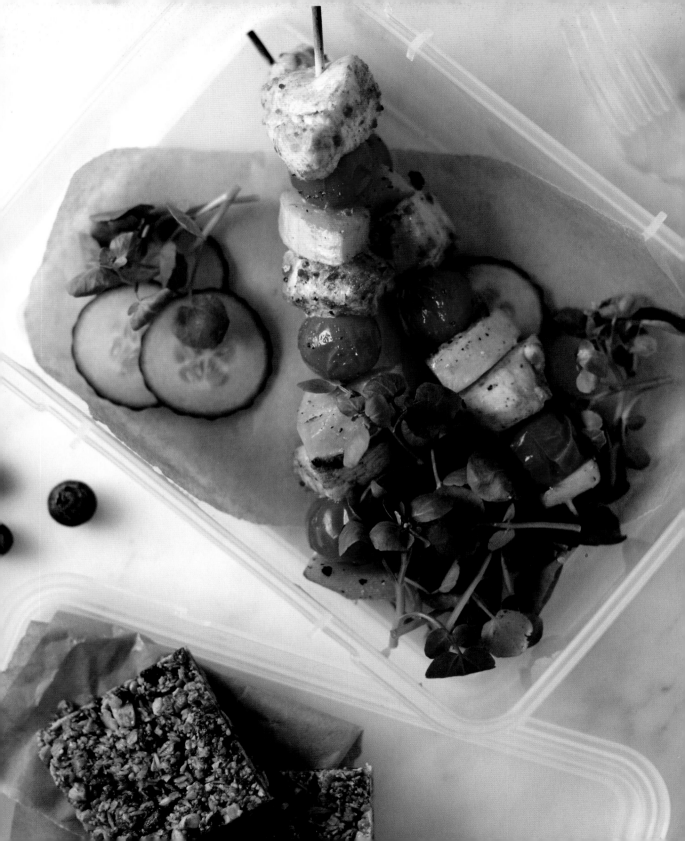

Quick lunches

It can be a struggle to find healthy food to eat on the go. Here are some yummy alternatives to the standard sandwich or wrap—simple, portable kebabs, soups, and salads that not only taste great, but will fill you up, too.

Taco lettuce wrap 4 ways

This is a skinny version of a wrap, using crisp romaine or Boston lettuce instead of a starchy taco or tortilla. For a packed lunch, simply wrap the filled lettuce leaves in plastic wrap or foil, as you would a sandwich.

1. Salmon and avocado

Serves 1

1 avocado
4 outer leaves from Boston lettuce or romaine
100g smoked salmon
Squeeze of lemon juice
1 tsp sesame seeds

Mash the avocado and dollop it into the base of the lettuce leaves. Add a strip of smoked salmon, a squeeze of lemon, a grinding of black pepper, and scatter with the sesame seeds.

- **CALORIES** 470
- PROTEIN 26G
- FAT 50G
- FIBER 7G
- CARBS 5G

2. Tuna and tomato salsa

Serves 1

3 oz canned tuna, drained
2 tomatoes, finely diced
¼ red onion, finely diced
Dash of Tabasco
Squeeze of lime juice
4 outer leaves from Boston
  lettuce or romaine
Handful of cilantro,
  chopped

Mix the tuna in a bowl with the tomatoes, red onion, Tabasco, lime juice, and some black pepper. Divide the mixture among the 4 lettuce leaves. Garnish with cilantro.

- **CALORIES** 140
- PROTEIN 26G
- FAT 2G
- FIBER 3G
- CARBS 7G

3. Feta and avocado bash

Serves 1

1 avocado
1 oz feta
Squeeze of lime juice
4 outer leaves from Boston
  lettuce or romaine
Handful of parsley, chopped

Place the avocado and feta in a bowl and use a fork or potato masher to blend them together, then stir in the lime juice. Divide the mixture among the 4 lettuce leaves, season with freshly ground black pepper, and sprinkle with the parsley.

- **CALORIES** 370
- PROTEIN 8G
- FAT 35G
- FIBER 6G
- CARBS 5G

4. Roast peppers with hummus and nuts

Serves 1

3 strips roasted red
  pepper from a jar, chopped
2 heaping tbsp hummus
4 outer leaves from Boston
  lettuce or romaine
2 tsp pine nuts

Mix the strips of pepper with the hummus in a bowl. Season with a pinch of salt and black pepper. Divide the mixture among the 4 lettuce leaves and sprinkle with the pine nuts.

- **CALORIES** 190
- PROTEIN 7G
- FAT 15G
- FIBER 2G
- CARBS 10G

Instant salads

Many people now take a salad in a plastic container to work for their lunch. The salads below all work well assembled in advance. Find a small container for the dressing (with a good lid so it doesn't leak!) and store the salad in a separate container to keep it crisp and fresh.

Lentil and feta salad

Lentils are a key part of the Mediterranean diet, containing plenty of fiber and protein to help keep you feeling fuller for longer. They are also a good source of iron.

Serves 2

¾ cup plus 2 tbsp canned, rinsed,
  and drained black or green lentils
1 spring onion, finely sliced
2 oz feta or Cheddar, crumbled
Handful of parsley, chopped
Handful of salad leaves, such as
  arugula or romaine
½ tsp dried herbs, such as thyme
  or oregano
Pinch of red pepper flakes

For the dressing:
1 tbsp balsamic vinegar
2 tbsp extra-virgin olive oil

Mix the lentils, spring onion, feta, parsley, salad leaves, dried herbs, and red pepper flakes in a bowl, and season to taste. Whisk together the oil and vinegar to make the dressing and drizzle it over the salad.

Tip: if preparing for one, the second portion will keep in the fridge for a couple of days.

- **CALORIES 190**
- PROTEIN 7G
- FAT 14G
- FIBER 3G
- CARBS 11G

Greek salad

The ultimate in Mediterranean-style food, a Greek salad makes a perfect light lunch, and also works well as a side dish for a main meal. Buy the very best vegetables you can—ripe tomatoes, good olives, fresh mint—and ideally serve at room temperature to get the most out of their flavors.

Serves 2

4 medium, vine-ripened tomatoes, chopped
½ cucumber, seeded and coarsely chopped
½ red onion, thinly sliced
8 black olives, pitted and halved
2 oz feta, diced
Handful of mint leaves, chopped

For the dressing:
2 tbsp extra-virgin olive oil
Juice of half a lemon
½ tsp dried oregano

Toss the tomatoes, cucumber, onion, olives, feta, and mint in a bowl. Whisk together the dressing ingredients and drizzle it over the salad. Summer holiday on a plate.

- **CALORIES** 190
- PROTEIN 5G
- FAT 15G
- FIBER 3G
- CARBS 10G

Tuna, artichoke, and butter bean salad

Artichokes are not only tasty, they are packed with wonderful nutrients and phytochemicals. They are so good for your gut bacteria that they are known as prebiotics.

Serves 2

3 oz canned tuna, drained
2 spring onions, chopped
8 cherry tomatoes, halved
1¾ cups canned butter beans, rinsed and drained
2 artichoke hearts from a jar, quartered

For the dressing:
2 tbsp olive oil
Juice of half a lemon
1 tsp Dijon mustard
Handful of parsley leaves, chopped

Place the tuna in a bowl and break it up into chunks. Add the spring onions, tomatoes, beans, and artichokes and toss everything together. Whisk together the dressing ingredients and drizzle it over the salad.

Tip: olive oil, like avocados and most nuts, contains large amounts of oleic acid and is a health-promoting staple of the Mediterranean diet. Enjoy it. Drizzle it on your salads, over hummus, on vegetables, beans, and legumes . . .

- **CALORIES** 410
- PROTEIN 40G
- FAT 16G
- FIBER 10G
- CARBS 30G

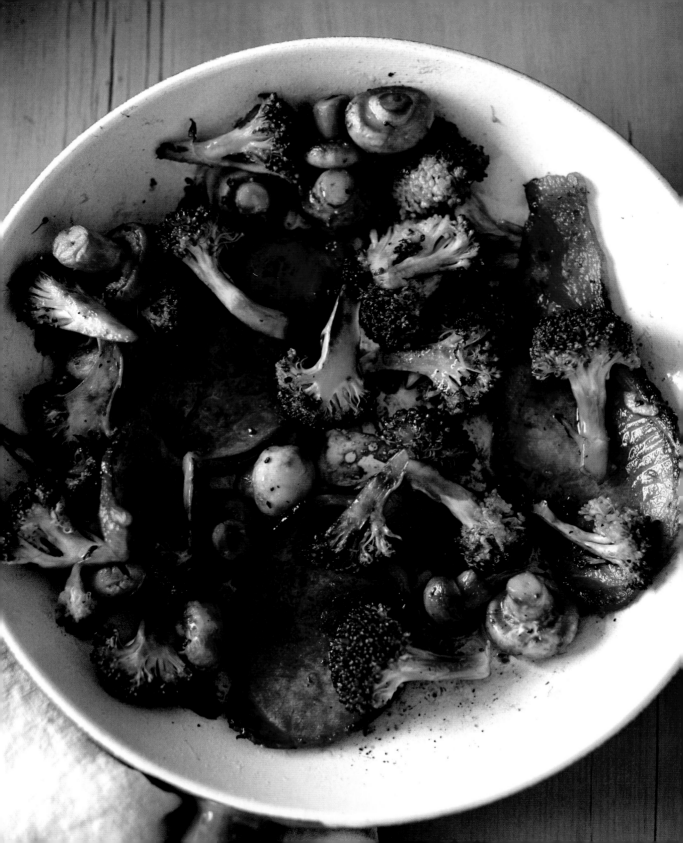

Dr. David Unwin's quick bacon and broccoli fry-up

A delicious, easy lunch, kindly sent to us by the inspirational GP Dr. David Unwin, who has been championing the low-carb, higher-fat approach to eating for some years. He has helped many of his patients lose weight, improve their blood sugars, and reverse their diabetes; and was doing this at a time when people didn't believe it was possible.

Serves 1

3 slices bacon, diced
1 tbsp olive oil
4 oz button mushrooms
7 oz broccoli, coarsely
  chopped, or leeks, sliced
½ oz cheese, grated

Fry the bacon in the olive oil, add the mushrooms and then the broccoli and cook until everything has softened and melded together. Add some black pepper and sprinkle on the cheese, and dig in. (Even better, if you have time: place the mixture in an oven dish under the broiler until it's golden brown on top.)

Tip: you can replace the bacon with either 2 oz halloumi, fried first like the bacon, or 3 oz peppered mackerel, which should be added at the end to the softened vegetable mixture.

- **CALORIES** 430
- PROTEIN 29G
- FAT 33G
- FIBER 6G
- CARBS 4G

Speedy spicy beans

This vegetarian dish—inspired by a recipe from Hashimoto on the Blood Sugar Diet website—is fabulously easy to make and is ready in 5 minutes.

Serves 1

½ red onion or shallot,
  chopped
½ tbsp olive oil
½ red bell pepper,
  seeded and chopped
½ medium zucchini, diced
  into ¾ inch pieces
1 garlic clove, chopped
  or crushed
1 chile, seeded and
  sliced, or 1 tsp red pepper
  flakes
8 oz reduced-sugar
  canned baked beans
Splash of Worcestershire
  sauce (optional)

In a medium pan, sweat the onion in the oil for a few minutes. Add the bell pepper, zucchini, garlic, and chile, and cook for another few minutes until the vegetables have slightly softened. Stir in the baked beans and Worcestershire sauce and make sure everything is thoroughly heated through before serving.

Tip: on a non-fast day you could add a slice of the seeded spelt and rye bread (see page 181).

- **CALORIES** 250
- PROTEIN 12G
- FAT 7G
- FIBER 9G
- CARBS 37G

Green beans with halloumi

A wonderfully crisp, green summer dish, which is also infinitely adaptable.

Serves 2

3 oz halloumi cheese,
  or 4 slices bacon,
  chopped
1 tbsp olive oil
½ lb green beans or other
  seasonal vegetables such
  as sugar snap peas,
  trimmed and diced
1 tbsp pecorino
  or Parmesan, grated
Handful of pine nuts
  or other seeds, toasted

Fry the halloumi in the oil. Steam, boil, or microwave the beans so they are still a bit crunchy. In a bowl, mix the hot beans with the halloumi and the pecorino. Season with black pepper and sprinkle with the pine nuts before serving.

- **CALORIES** 320
- PROTEIN 17G
- FAT 26G
- FIBER 3G
- CARBS 6G

Omelet 2 ways

1. Japanese omelet

Serves 1

2 eggs
½ tbsp soy sauce
2 oz cabbage or greens,
 finely chopped (or use
 leftover greens)
1 tbsp coconut oil or light
 olive oil
½ tsp finely chopped
 fresh ginger
¼ tsp red pepper flakes
2-3 spring onions, finely
 diced
Small handful of cilantro
 leaves, chopped
Sushi pickled ginger from
 a jar (optional)

Whisk the eggs with the soy sauce. Steam, microwave, or boil the greens for a couple of minutes, so they are tender but still crisp. In a small frying pan, heat the oil and add the ginger, red pepper flakes, and spring onions. Fry gently for about a minute, then pour in the eggs. Immediately add the greens and cilantro and cook the omelet gently until the underside is golden brown. Fold it in half and serve it while it is still a bit runny, with sushi pickled ginger, if using, and a grating of black pepper.

- **CALORIES** 270
- PROTEIN 14G
- FAT 21G
- FIBER 2G
- CARBS 5G

2. Cheese and asparagus omelet

This is Michael's absolute favorite, sprinkled liberally with red pepper flakes for an extra kick.

Serves 1

3-4 asparagus spears,
 halved lengthwise and cut
 into 1½ inch pieces
Pat of butter
2 eggs, beaten
½ oz sharp Cheddar, grated
1 teaspoon grated Parmesan
Pinch of red pepper flakes
 (optional)

Steam the asparagus for 1½ minutes (or less if using a microwave). In a small nonstick frying pan, melt the butter, then pour in the eggs and cook them over a gentle heat. Scatter the Cheddar and Parmesan over the surface and add the asparagus. When the surface is still a little bit soft, fold the omelet in half. Season and sprinkle with red pepper flakes, if using.

- **CALORIES** 290
- PROTEIN 23G
- FAT 22G
- FIBER 1G
- CARBS 1G

Kebabs to go

These make delicious, healthy snacks on a stick. With a bit of planning you can have them ready to take to work. Buy a pack of short wooden skewers that fit into your lunch box. For kebabs made of meat or fish, it would be wise to include a small ice pack in the box if you are going to be out for more than an hour or two in the heat.

In the ideal world you would cook them over a barbecue, but they still taste superb done under a hot broiler or on a griddle.

1. Lemon shrimp kebabs

Serves 1

2 tbsp olive oil
Juice of 1 lemon
12 jumbo shrimp, fresh or frozen and thawed
12 cherry tomatoes
3 asparagus spears, cut into 4 pieces
3 wooden skewers, soaked in water

Place the oil in a bowl, mix in the lemon juice, and season well with salt and plenty of black pepper. Then add the shrimp, tomatoes, and asparagus and toss everything so it gets a good coating. Thread the shrimp and vegetables onto the skewers and place them under a hot broiler for 10 minutes, turning frequently. Serve with a dollop of Greek yogurt (adds 30 calories).

- **CALORIES** 360
- PROTEIN 21G
- FAT 28G
- FIBER 3G
- CARBS 7G

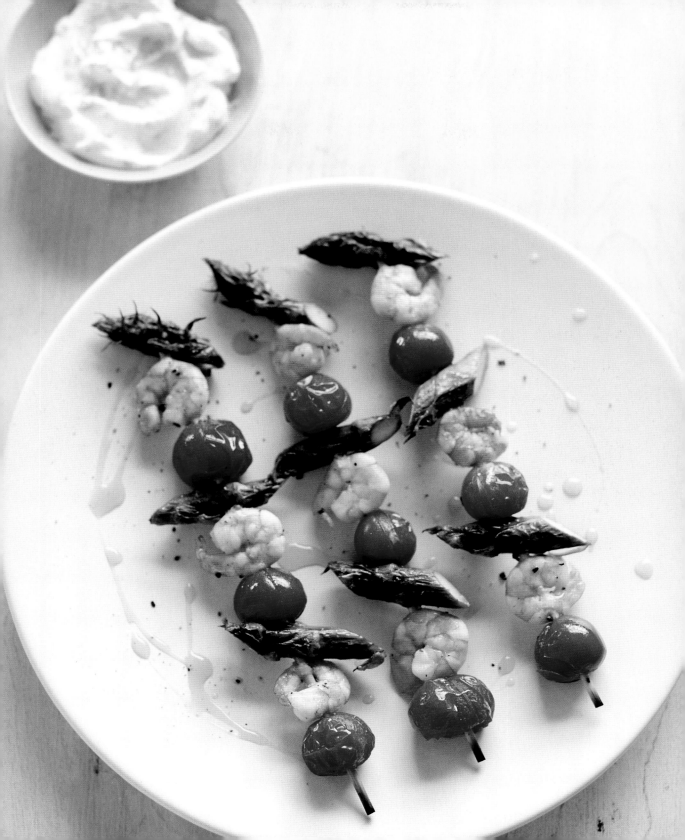

2. Halloumi kebabs

Serves 1

3½ oz halloumi
6 artichoke hearts from
  a jar
1 red bell pepper
2 tbsp olive oil
1 tsp ras el hanout or
  paprika
3 wooden skewers, soaked
  in water

Dice the halloumi into 9 cubes, halve the artichoke hearts, and chop the bell pepper into 12 pieces. Put them in a bowl with the oil and ras el hanout and some seasoning, and toss everything well so it gets a good coating. Thread the kebab pieces onto the skewers, then place them under a hot broiler for 5 to 6 minutes, turning frequently. Serve with low-sugar sweet chili sauce (see page 175) or raita (see page 72).

- **CALORIES** 430
- PROTEIN 19G
- FAT 34G
- FIBER 3G
- CARBS 15G

3. Ploughman's on a stick

I like to think of this as a tasty low-carb version of what you might get in a pub. Choose your favorite cheese—just make sure it is not too runny or crumbly, so that it stays on the stick. For variation, you could add rolled slices of salami or ham.

Serves 1

3 slices of ham, cut into
  strips and rolled
9 pickled cocktail onions
  or small gherkins
1 apple, cored and chopped
  into chunks
2 oz Cheddar, diced
3 wooden skewers
1 tbsp coarsely chopped
  pickle

Thread the ham, onions, apple, and cheese onto the skewers. Serve with the pickle.

- **CALORIES** 400
- PROTEIN 24G
- FAT 25G
- FIBER 2G
- CARBS 18G

4. Spiced lamb kebabs

Serves 1

4 oz lamb, chops or leg
1 green bell pepper, seeded
2 tbsp olive oil
2 tsp harissa paste or curry
 paste
12 button mushrooms
3 wooden skewers,
 soaked in water

Dice the lamb and bell pepper into 12 pieces. Pour the oil into a bowl and stir in the harissa paste. Add the lamb and mix well. If you have time, leave it to marinate for a few hours. Then add the bell pepper and mushrooms and stir well so everything gets a good coating. Thread the kebab pieces onto the skewers, alternating the lamb, bell pepper, and mushrooms. Place them under a hot grill for 10 minutes, turning frequently. Serve with raita or tzatziki (see page 72).

- **CALORIES** 460
- PROTEIN 32G
- FAT 45G
- FIBER 5G
- CARBS 8G

5. Paprika chicken kebab

Serves 1

1 boneless, skinless chicken
 breast
1 tbsp olive oil, plus a little
 extra for drizzling
1 garlic clove, crushed
1 tsp paprika
Juice of half a lemon
Pinch of red pepper flakes
 (optional)
1 zucchini
1 red onion, quartered
3 wooden skewers, soaked
 in water

Slice the chicken breast into 3 long strips and then dice each strip, aiming to get about 12 cubes. Mix the oil in a bowl with the garlic, paprika, lemon juice, red pepper flakes, if using, and some seasoning, and then add the chicken, tossing everything together so it gets a good coating. Chop the zucchini into 12 chunks and then cut the onion quarters into thirds so you have 12 chunks of that, too. Toss the zucchini and onion in a bowl with a drizzle of oil and some salt and pepper.

Thread the kebab pieces onto the skewers, alternating the chicken, zucchini, and onion. Place them under a hot broiler for 12 to 15 minutes, turning every 3 to 4 minutes. Serve with tzatziki (see page 72).

- **CALORIES** 190
- PROTEIN 12G
- FAT 14G
- FIBER 1G
- CARBS 6G

6. Piri piri chicken sticks

Serves 1

1 boneless, skinless chicken
  breast
2 tbsp olive oil
1 tsp piri piri seasoning
12 cherry tomatoes
¼ butternut squash, peeled
  and cubed (or 12 pieces
  of chopped store-bought)
3 wooden skewers, soaked
  in water

Slice the chicken breast into 3 long strips and then dice each strip, aiming to get 12 cubes. Mix 1 tbsp of the oil and the piri piri seasoning in a bowl, then add the chicken, tossing it well so it gets a good coating. Leave it to marinate for a few hours, if time permits.

Toss the tomatoes and butternut squash in a separate bowl with the remaining 1 tbsp oil and some salt and pepper. Thread the kebab pieces onto the skewers, alternating the chicken, tomato, and squash. Place them under a hot grill for 12 to 15 minutes, turning every 3 to 4 minutes. Serve with raita (see page 72).

Tip: to make your own piri piri flavoring, mix together 1 tsp paprika, 1 tsp oregano, 1 to 2 fresh chiles, seeded and diced (or 1 to 2 tsp red pepper flakes), and 1 tsp garlic, either paste or a finely chopped clove.

- **CALORIES** 360
- PROTEIN 13G
- FAT 28G
- FIBER 4G
- CARBS 18G

7. Chinese tofu kebabs

Serves 1

4 oz tofu
2 spring onions
1 red bell pepper, seeded
1 tbsp olive oil
Juice of half a lime
1 tsp Chinese 5-spice
1 tsp soy sauce
1 tsp fish sauce
3 wooden skewers, soaked
  in water

Dice the tofu into 12 cubes, cut each spring onion into 6 pieces and the bell pepper into 12. Mix the oil in a bowl with the lime juice, spice, soy and fish sauce and then add the tofu, spring onions, and bell pepper, tossing everything well so it gets a good coating. Thread the skewers, alternating ingredients, and place them under a hot grill for 10 minutes, turning frequently. Serve with low-sugar sweet chili sauce (see page 175).

- **CALORIES** 230
- PROTEIN 12G
- FAT 16G
- FIBER 3G
- CARBS 12G

8. Satay chicken kebabs

An exotic South East Asian mix. Irresistible.

Serves 2

2 boneless, skinless chicken
  breasts
1 garlic clove, crushed
½ red chile, seeded and
  chopped
2 tbsp soy sauce
1 tbsp coconut oil
6 wooden skewers, soaked
  in water

For the satay sauce:
2 tbsp coconut oil
2 spring onions, diced
1 garlic clove, crushed
½ red chile, seeded and
  chopped
3 tbsp peanut butter
½ tbsp fish sauce
½ cup coconut milk

To make the kebabs, slice each chicken breast into 3 long strips and then dice each strip, aiming to get 12 to 15 cubes from each. Make a marinade in a bowl by mixing the garlic, chile, soy sauce, and oil. Toss the chicken pieces in the marinade, making sure they are well coated. Cover them with plastic wrap and leave them in the fridge overnight.

When you are ready to eat, thread 4 or 5 cubes onto each wooden skewer, season them with salt and pepper, and place them under a hot broiler for 12 to 15 minutes, turning every 3 to 4 minutes.

Meanwhile, to make the sauce, put a pan on medium heat, add the oil, and sauté the spring onions, garlic, and chile for 3 to 4 minutes, or until they are soft. Add the peanut butter and fish sauce and keep stirring for another 2 minutes. Transfer the mixture to a food processor, add the coconut milk, and blend to a smooth paste.

Taste the sauce and add a splash of soy sauce if you wish. Serve the kebabs on a bed of arugula with the dipping sauce on the side.

- **CALORIES** 460
- PROTEIN 33G
- FAT 44G
- FIBER 2G
- CARBS 10G

Soups

Soup not only makes a delicious meal, it can be very filling. Studies have shown that eating food blended into a soup keeps you satisfied for longer, compared with eating the same food separately along with the extra fluid. We suggest making enough for 4 portions so that you can put anything left over in the freezer for instant sustenance another day.

Celeriac and apple soup

Serves 4

1 tbsp olive oil
1 onion, chopped
1 leek, sliced
¾-inch fresh ginger,
  chopped
1 celeriac (celery root),
  peeled and chopped
4 apples, cored and
  quartered
Large pinch of dried thyme
2 quarts vegetable or
  chicken stock
¾ cup crème fraîche
1 tbsp nuts, chopped

Heat the oil in a large saucepan. Add the onion, leek, and ginger and cook over medium heat for 10 minutes, until they are soft. Stir in the celeriac, apples, and thyme and cook for a few more minutes. Pour in the stock and some seasoning and simmer for 30 minutes. When the celeriac is tender, remove the soup from the heat and use an immersion blender (or a food processor) to blitz it until it is smooth. Stir in half the crème fraîche, reserving the remainder to dollop into each bowl. Serve with a scattering of nuts.

- CALORIES 320
- PROTEIN 5G
- FAT 24G
- FIBER 8G
- CARBS 20G

Chicken lime laksa

Serves 4

Bunch of fresh cilantro
Drizzle of olive oil
4 spring onions, sliced
1 red bell pepper, seeded
  and sliced
1 tsp chili paste
1 tsp ginger paste
1 tsp Chinese 5-spice
11-12 oz chopped butternut
  squash
5¼ cups chicken or
  vegetable stock
Juice of 2 limes
1 tbsp soy sauce
1 tbsp Thai fish sauce
11-12 oz cooked chicken,
  diced
14 oz green beans
1½ cups canned coconut
  milk
2 large handfuls of baby
  spinach leaves, or fresh
  greens, chopped

Chop off the cilantro stalks, retaining the leaves. Heat the oil in a large saucepan and fry the stalks, spring onions, bell pepper, chili paste, ginger paste, and Chinese 5 spice on medium heat for 2 to 3 minutes. Add the butternut squash and cook for another 2 minutes, then pour in the stock, lime juice, soy and fish sauces and bring the mixture to a boil. Turn down the heat and simmer for 10 minutes. Add the chicken, beans, coconut milk, and spinach and cook until the beans have softened and the chicken has warmed through. Serve topped with the cilantro leaves.

- **CALORIES** 330
- PROTEIN 21G
- FAT 23G
- FIBER 2G
- CARBS 9G

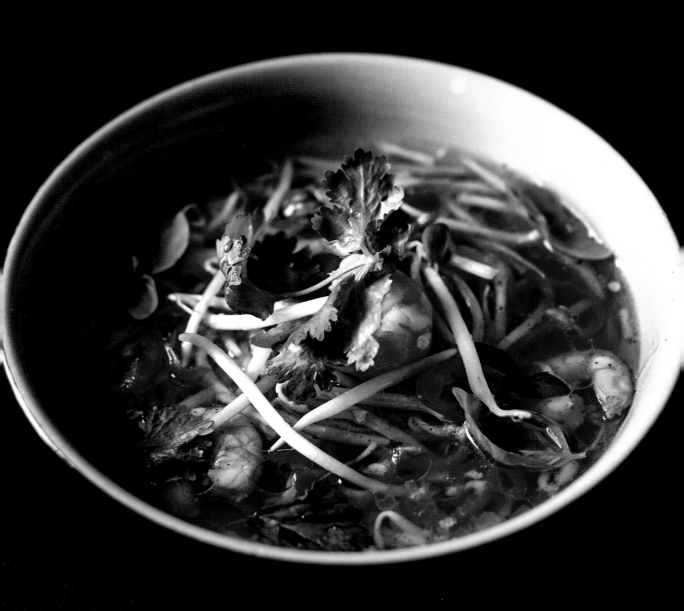

Vietnamese pho

This soup makes a wonderful light lunch. The low-carb konjac noodles add few calories to the dish. They are made from yams and have been eaten in Japan for centuries.

Serves 2

2 tsp coconut oil
¾-inch fresh ginger, grated
2 spring onions, chopped
1 quart vegetable stock
Juice of 1 lime
1 tbsp Thai fish sauce
1 tbsp mirin or cider vinegar
8 large shrimp (fresh or
  frozen)
1 (12-oz) bag of bean
  sprouts
2 to 3 spring greens,
  shredded
4 oz konjac noodles,
  rinsed and drained
  (optional, see tip)
Handful of fresh basil
  or cilantro
½ red chile, seeded and
  finely sliced, or pinch of
  red pepper flakes

Heat the oil in a large saucepan, and fry the ginger and spring onions for 2 to 3 minutes. Pour in the stock, add the lime juice, fish sauce, and mirin and season with salt and pepper. Bring the mixture to a boil and simmer for 10 minutes. Add the shrimp and cook them for 5 minutes more, or until they turn pink. Then add the bean sprouts, greens, and konjac noodles, if using. Serve the pho with the herbs and red pepper flakes scattered over the top.

Tip: if konjac noodles are not available, you might substitute 4 oz of spaghetti squash (see page 107), or skip them altogether as the bean sprouts provide plenty of texture. You can also replace the shrimp with tofu, chicken, or beef.

- **CALORIES** 120
- PROTEIN 13G
- FAT 7G
- FIBER 2G
- CARBS 7G

Tomato, ham, and lentil soup

A favorite, comforting soup, often to be found bubbling away when we visit Michael's mum.

Serves 4

2 tbsp olive oil
1 onion, chopped
1 red bell pepper, seeded and chopped
1 garlic clove, crushed
1 tsp red pepper flakes
6 oz red lentils
2 (14-oz) cans chopped tomatoes
6⅓ cups vegetable or chicken stock
7 oz leftover ham (or bacon or pancetta), chopped
2 tbsp parsley or cilantro, chopped
7-8 oz container sour cream and chive dip (full-fat)

Heat the oil in a large saucepan and gently fry the onion and bell pepper for 6 to 8 minutes. Add the garlic and red pepper flakes and stir for a minute, then pour in the lentils, tomatoes, and stock. Bring the pan to a boil, cover and simmer for 30 minutes, or until the lentils are really tender and beginning to break up. Stir in the ham and parsley and season to taste, then remove the soup from the heat and mash it coarsely with a potato masher, leaving some texture. Serve each portion with 1 tbsp of the sour cream and chive dip.

- **CALORIES** 440
- PROTEIN 25G
- FAT 23G
- FIBER 5G
- CARBS 40G

Miso soup

Miso soup is made from fermented soy beans with a base of dashi, a Japanese broth of seaweed and dried fish. Michael lived on this (without any of the extras), when he did a 4-day fast prior to starting the 5:2 Fast Diet. He found it a lifeline and looked forward to it—warm and tasty and very low in calories.

Serves 1

1 cup plus 2 tbsp dashi stock
2 tbsp miso paste
1 spring onion, finely chopped
¼-inch fresh ginger, grated
1 tbsp mirin

Mix 1 tbsp dashi stock with the miso paste to dissolve it. Heat the remaining stock in a saucepan and stir in the loosened paste, bring it to a boil, and allow it to simmer for 10 minutes. Add the spring onion and ginger and simmer for another 2 to 3 minutes.

For a more substantial version, choose a handful of any of the following, each about 10 calories, unless stated: Chinese cabbage, bok choy, broccoli, any leafy green vegetable, canned water chestnuts, bamboo shoots, bean sprouts, grated or spiralized carrot, finely chopped leeks, or shiitake mushrooms (adds 20 calories for these). Simmer the vegetables in the stock for about 5 minutes, depending on how crunchy you like them.

For a shot of protein, you could also add: a raw egg, cracked in to poach for 3 to 5 minutes; or 2 oz any cooked fish or meat, such as pork, turkey, chicken, poached salmon, or crab (adds 90 calories); or 4 oz tempeh, tofu, or shrimp (adds approximately 100 calories).

For a more exotic option, top with kaiso (dried seaweed, which rehydrates in hot liquid) or nori (shredded seaweed). You could also add a little sushi pickled ginger from a jar.

- **CALORIES** 90
- PROTEIN 6G
- FAT 3G
- FIBER 0G
- CARBS 11G

Roasted red pepper and squash soup

Serves 4

4 red or orange bell
 peppers, halved and
 seeded
½ large butternut squash,
 peeled and diced (or
 ¾-1 lb bag chopped
 squash)
1 onion, diced
2 tbsp olive oil
1 quart vegetable stock
½ tsp red pepper flakes,
 or ½ red chile, seeded
 and diced
Handful of parsley or
 cilantro, chopped

Preheat the oven to 350°F. Spread the bell peppers, butternut squash, and onion on a large oven pan. Season them and drizzle with 1 tbsp of the oil. Bake the vegetables until the edges begin to blacken (about 20 minutes). When the bell peppers have cooled sufficiently, remove most of the skin and coarsely chop them.

Heat the remaining 1 tbsp oil in a large saucepan and put in the baked vegetables. Add the stock and red pepper flakes and bring it to a boil, then let it simmer for about 20 minutes, or until everything is soft. Remove the pan from the heat and blend the soup with an immersion blender or food processor. Bring it back to a boil before serving it garnished with the parsley. (For a richer dish, you can add a handful of fried chorizo; alternatively, add 1 tbsp each of fried diced halloumi or toasted nuts—see page 177.)

- **CALORIES** 150
- PROTEIN 3G
- FAT 6G
- FIBER 4G
- CARBS 22G

Gazpacho

A simple summer classic.

Serves 4

2 (14-oz) cans chopped
 tomatoes
½ cucumber, seeded and
 cut into chunks
1 garlic clove, minced
1 red bell pepper, seeded
 and chopped
2 tbsp olive oil, plus more
 to drizzle
3 tbsp cider vinegar or red
 wine vinegar
Handful of basil leaves,
 shredded
12 ice cubes

Put the tomatoes in a food processor, followed by the cucumber, garlic, bell pepper, oil, vinegar, and most of the basil. Season with salt and freshly ground black pepper. Add a few ice cubes, a drizzle of oil, and a sprinkling of basil to each bowl before serving.

- **CALORIES** 100
- PROTEIN 3G
- FAT 5G
- FIBER 8G
- CARBS 10G

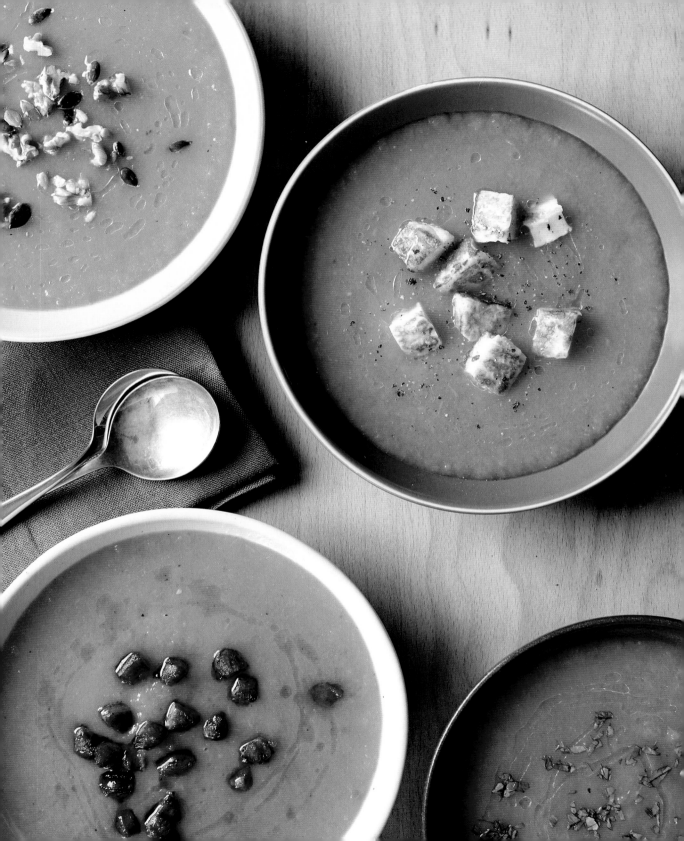

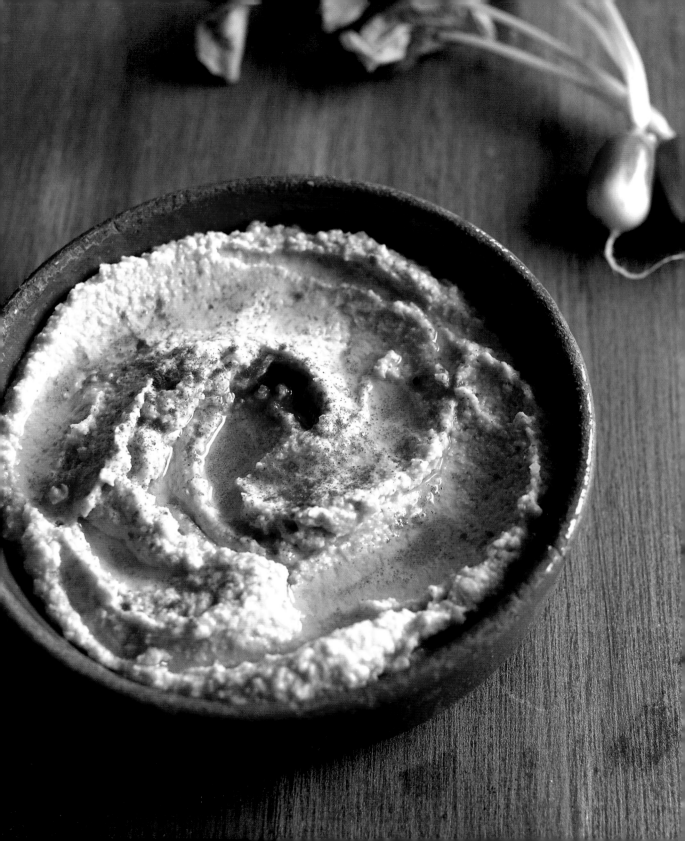

Smart snacks

A range of tasty, filling dips and nibbles that will have minimal impact on blood sugars.

Skinny dips

The following dips can be served as accompaniments to almost any meal. For a light lunch, have a portion with batons (sticks) or chunks of any crunchy, salad-type vegetable as a delicious alternative to crisps, bread, and pita.

Perfect hummus

Makes 4 portions

*1 (14-oz) can chickpeas,
  rinsed and drained*
*3 tbsp lemon juice
  (or more, to taste)*
*6 tbsp extra-virgin olive oil,
  plus more to drizzle*
4 tsp tahini
2 garlic cloves, crushed
1 tsp ground cumin
Pinch of salt
3 tbsp water, as required
1 tsp paprika

Blend the chickpeas, lemon juice, oil, tahini, garlic, cumin, salt, and water in a food processor until you have a creamy puree. Serve it with a drizzle of oil and a sprinkling of paprika.

- **CALORIES** 210
- PROTEIN 9G
- FAT 13G
- FIBER 5G
- CARBS 17G

Tzatziki

Makes 4 portions

2 small cucumbers
1 cup plus 2 tbsp full-fat
  Greek yogurt
Juice of 1 lemon
2-3 garlic cloves, finely
  grated
1 tbsp olive oil
1 tsp paprika

Peel and seed the cucumbers, then grate or finely dice them. Combine them in a bowl with the yogurt, lemon juice, garlic, oil, paprika, and a pinch of salt and pepper.

- **CALORIES** 140
- PROTEIN 4G
- FAT 1G
- FIBER 0G
- CARBS 4G

Raita

This makes a great dip, as well as a tasty accompaniment to a curry.

Makes 4 portions

½ cucumber
1 cup full-fat Greek
  yogurt
¼ tsp cumin seeds
2-3 mint leaves, finely
  chopped

Peel and seed the cucumber, then grate or finely dice it. Combine it in a bowl with the yogurt, cumin seeds, mint leaves, and a large pinch of salt.

- **CALORIES** 80
- PROTEIN 4G
- FAT 6G
- FIBER 0G
- CARBS 2G

Smoked fish paté

Makes 2 portions

1 smoked mackerel or trout
 fillet
3 tbsp full-fat cream cheese
Squeeze of lemon juice
1-2 tsp hot horseradish
 sauce
½ cucumber, thickly sliced

Remove the skin from the mackerel fillet and mash the fish in a bowl with the cream cheese and lemon juice. Season the mixture with black pepper, and add the horseradish sauce, to taste. Serve the paté on the slices of cucumber (or on seeded crackers—see page 75) or with vegetable batons as a dip.

- **CALORIES** 270
- PROTEIN 14G
- FAT 23G
- FIBER 0G
- CARBS 3G

Guacamole

Perfect as a dip or as a side dish to add a bit of zing to a meal.

Makes 2 portions

1 ripe avocado, coarsely
 mashed
½ chile, seeded and
 finely chopped, or red
 pepper flakes to taste
Juice of half a lime (or
 lemon)
2 large slices beefsteak
 tomato

Mash the avocado in a bowl with the chile, lime juice, and some seasoning. Spread the guacamole on a couple of slices of tomato, or serve it with vegetable batons as a dip.

- **CALORIES** 140
- PROTEIN 3G
- FAT 28G
- FIBER 5G
- CARBS 5G

Why nuts make the ideal snack

For many years we've been wary of nuts because of their high fat and calorie content. Big mistake! Lots of studies have shown that eating a small handful of nuts a day actually helps you lose weight and cuts the risk of heart disease. Nuts are a key ingredient of the Mediterranean diet and, although it is true that they are fairly high in calories, your body finds them hard to digest and consequently many of those calories are not absorbed.

Packed with protein, fiber, and healthy essential fats, they keep you full without significantly increasing your blood sugars, and contribute to the good bacteria in your gut, too. Go for salt-free nuts if you can, because you are less likely to overeat with them.

Savory Brazil nut butter

Makes 4 portions

6 oz Brazil nuts, soaked in water for 24 hours, rinsed and drained
2–3 garlic cloves
3 tbsp lemon juice
4 tbsp rapeseed oil
2 tbsp tahini
Pinch of cayenne pepper

- CALORIES 110
- PROTEIN 2G
- FAT 12G
- FIBER 1G
- CARBS 1G

Blend the nuts, garlic, lemon juice, oil, tahini, and cayenne in a food processor until you have a smooth paste. Loosen it with a little water if necessary and season it with a pinch of salt and black pepper. Transfer it to a bowl, cover it with plastic wrap, and chill it in the fridge until you want to use it. Serve it with batons of carrots, celery, bell peppers, or cauliflower.

Healthy ploughman's

Cheese goes brilliantly with fruit such as apples or pears. It also works well with blackberries or blueberries. For a super-simple lunch snack, take a matchbox-size piece of hard cheese, an apple or pear, or a handful of berries, along with a stalk of celery and a couple of seeded crackers (see recipe below).

Thin seeded crackers

Perfect for eating with a dip or with cheese. These thin crackers contain lots of fiber and omega-3, and are an excellent source of heart-healthy, inflammation-reducing, essential fatty acids.

Makes 24 small crackers
(calories per cracker)

⅓ cup spelt flour
  (or any whole grain flour)
¼ cup cold water
1 heaping tsp Marmite
  (or yeast extract
  equivalent, optional)
¼ cup hot water
Extra flavoring, such
  as black pepper, chile,
  rosemary, or thyme
½ cup seeds made up of
  equal amounts of golden
  flaxseeds, chia seeds,
  sunflower seeds, and
  sesame seeds
¼ tsp sea salt

Preheat the oven to 300°F. In a medium bowl, mix the flour and ¼ cup cold water. In a separate bowl, dissolve the Marmite in ¼ cup hot water and pour it into the flour. Add extra flavoring or herbs, if using. Now stir in the seeds and the salt. Leave the dough to bind for 15 minutes, stirring occasionally.

Line a large baking sheet with parchment paper and brush oil liberally over the surface, or use a silicon baking pan or mat. Put the mixture onto the tray and spread it very thinly with the back of a fork, to about ⅛-inch thick. Sprinkle with a little extra salt and bake for about 20 minutes.

Then, using a knife, slice the baked dough into small crackers. Carefully remove them from the parchment paper and turn them over. Return them to the oven for another 15 minutes or so, until they start to turn golden. Turn the oven off but leave the crackers inside for another 15 to 30 minutes to let them dry out. They can be stored in an airtight container for up to a week.

Tip: make sure chia makes up a quarter of the seed mixture, as it helps to bind the crackers. The rest of the seeds can be adjusted according to taste.

- **CALORIES** 50
- PROTEIN 2G
- FAT 4G
- FIBER 1G
- CARBS 2G

Seedy bars

Made with wholesome, unprocessed nuts, seeds, fruit, and no added sugar, these seedy bars have a deliciously chewy texture.

Makes 24 small squares

½ cup plus 2 tbsp
  coconut oil
4 oz blueberries or figs,
  chopped
4 oz soft dates, finely
  chopped (about 15 large)
¼ cup jumbo oats
½ cup rolled oats
  (ideally with bran)
3 tbsp mixed seeds
  (sunflower, pumpkin,
  sesame, etc.)
3 tbsp hazelnuts or
  almonds, toasted and
  chopped
3 tbsp dried cranberries,
  goji berries, or raisins
Pinch of salt

Preheat the oven to 325°F and line a greased 8-inch square metal baking pan with parchment paper. In a food processor, blitz the oil, blueberries, and dates. Mix in the oats, seeds, nuts, dried fruit, and salt. Press the mixture down flat in the pan and bake it for about 30 minutes. Let the pan cool for 10 to 20 minutes, then cut into small squares before the bars set, and carefully lay them out on a rack to dry. They can be stored in an airtight container for a few days.

- CALORIES 80
- PROTEIN 2G
- FAT 4G
- FIBER 1G
- CARBS 10G

Parmesan crisps

A delicious and surprisingly healthy alternative to cheese straws. What's more, they take only 2 minutes to prepare and less than that to cook.

Makes 8 portions

4 oz Parmesan,
  finely grated
4 oz Cheddar, grated
4 oz ground almonds

Preheat the oven to 300°F and line a nonstick baking sheet with parchment paper. Mix the cheeses and almonds in a bowl, then, using a teaspoon, drop dollops of the mixture on the baking sheet. Bake them for 2 minutes, until they start to brown around the edges. Let them cool slightly and then dig in.

Tip: to prevent the paper on the baking sheet from curling up at the edges, hold it in place with a few blobs of strategically placed oil.

- CALORIES 180
- PROTEIN 10G
- FAT 15G
- FIBER 1G
- CARBS 1G

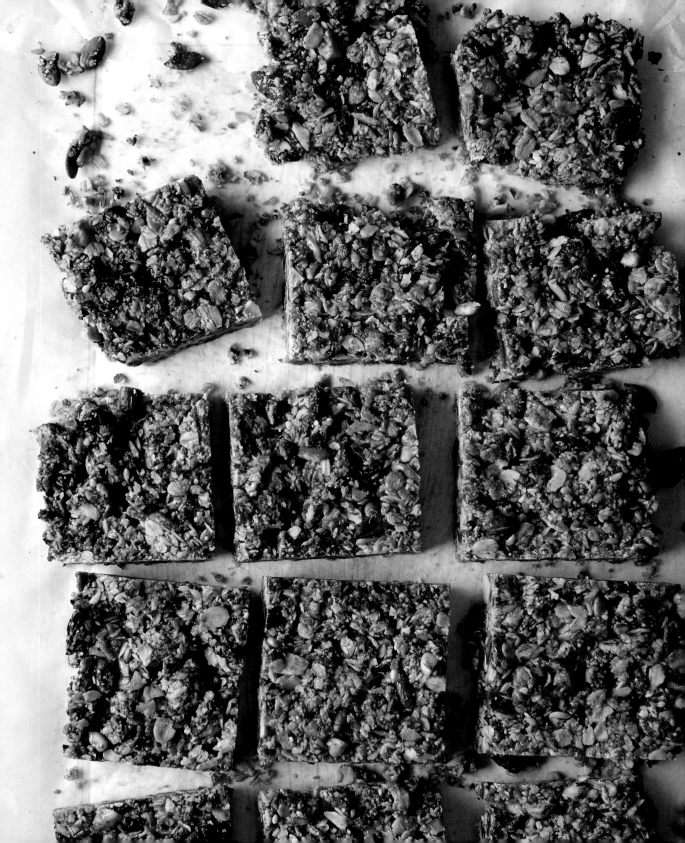

Easy Weekday Suppers

Simplicity and speed are the name of the game here. You will find many familiar favorites, lightly tweaked to replace starchy foods with delicious alternatives, and lots of other tasty and satisfying low-carb recipes that will help you lose weight and improve your blood sugars.

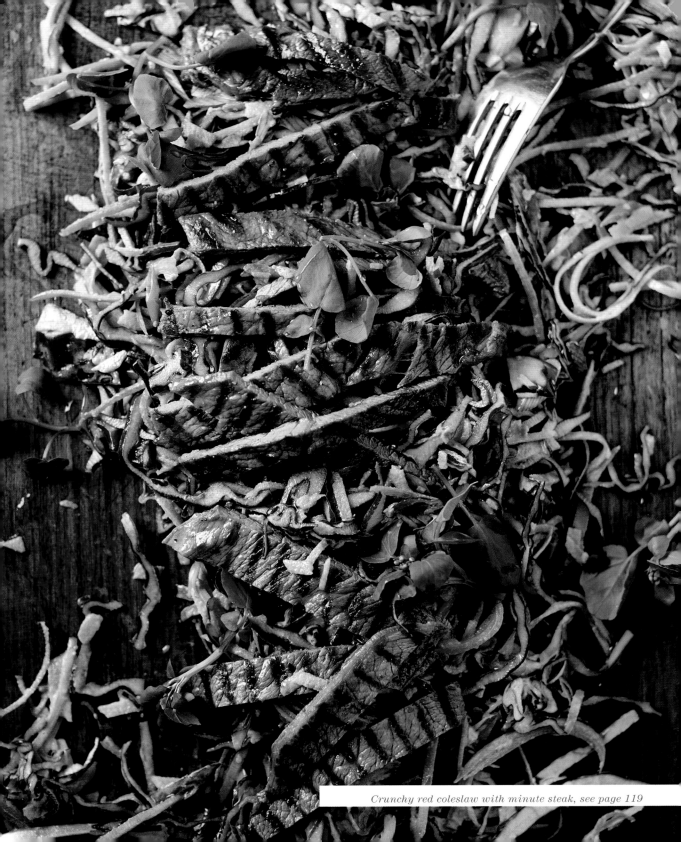

Crunchy red coleslaw with minute steak, see page 119

Roasted red pepper with anchovies

A scrumptious light supper, served here with quinoa or brown rice to mop up the juices.

Serves 1

1 red bell pepper
2-3 medium mushrooms,
  finely diced
1 tbsp pine nuts
1 garlic clove, finely
  chopped or crushed
6 cherry tomatoes, halved
1 tbsp olive oil
4 anchovies in oil
Handful of basil or
  cilantro leaves

Preheat the oven to 400°F. Cut the bell pepper in half, remove the stalk and seeds, and place the bell pepper in a baking dish. In a bowl, mix the mushrooms, pine nuts, garlic, and tomatoes, along with most of the olive oil. Spoon the mushroom mixture into the bell pepper halves. Lay the anchovies on top, drizzle with the remaining olive oil, and season with black pepper.

Bake the bell pepper for 20 to 25 minutes, or until some of the edges are slightly charred and the flesh has softened. Pour any juices in the dish over the bell pepper and garnish with basil. Serve with a salad of mixed leaves and arugula and 2 tbsp brown rice or quinoa (adds 35 calories).

- **CALORIES** 120
- PROTEIN 6G
- FAT 7G
- FIBER 3G
- CARBS 10G

Spicy spinach and lentils

A wonderful filling dahl, full of rich creamy flavors and surprisingly filling.

Serves 2

1 small onion, chopped
2 tbsp olive or coconut oil
2 garlic cloves, chopped
1-2 chiles, seeded and
  finely diced, or 1-2 tsp
  red pepper flakes
2 tsp cumin seeds
1 tsp ground cilantro
1 tsp turmeric (optional)
¾-inch fresh ginger, diced
Juice of half a lemon
1½ cups canned coconut
  milk
7 oz dry green lentils,
  rinsed, or 1 (14-oz) can
  green lentils, rinsed and
  drained
¾ cup water if using dry
  lentils (just a dash if using
  canned)
7-8 oz fresh spinach or
  frozen and thawed
Handful of cilantro,
  chopped

In a medium pan or casserole with a lid, gently fry the onion in the oil for 5 to 10 minutes. Stir in the garlic and cook for 1 minute more before adding the chiles, cumin seeds, turmeric (if using), and ginger. Cook for 2 minutes, then add the lemon juice, coconut milk, and lentils. Cover and simmer for 20 minutes (or for 5 minutes if using canned lentils), stirring occasionally and adding more water if needed. When the lentils are beginning to soften, add the spinach and cook for another 3 to 5 minutes. Season and serve with cilantro stirred through.

Tip: to make the dish more substantial you can add a handful of roasted cashew nuts, fried chicken, or paneer cheese; adjust the calories accordingly.

- **CALORIES** 320
- PROTEIN 7G
- FAT 26G
- FIBER 3G
- CARBS 14G

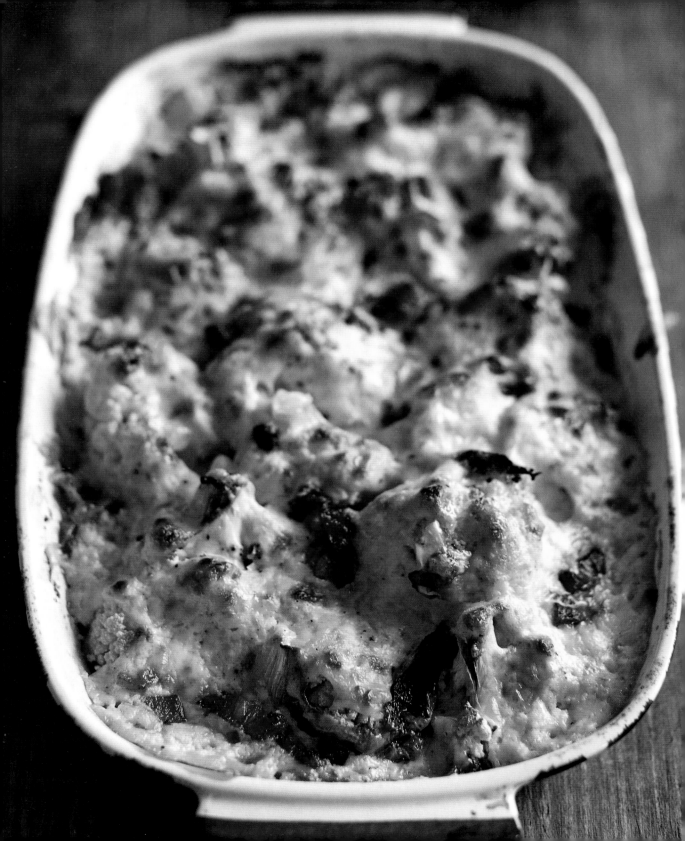

Cauliflower cheese

An old favorite with a low-carb, higher-fat twist. I enjoy munching jalapeños with mine, so have suggested mixing them in to give it a bit of a kick.

Serves 4

2 medium cauliflowers, broken into florets
7 oz ricotta
¾ cup crème fraîche
½ tbsp Worcestershire sauce
4 oz aged Cheddar, grated
2 oz diced bacon or lardons, fried (optional)
2-3 large jalapeño peppers from a jar, seeded and finely diced (optional)
2 oz Parmesan, grated

Preheat the oven to 325°F. Place the cauliflower florets in a baking dish in the oven. In a medium bowl, mix the ricotta, crème fraîche, Worcestershire sauce, and Cheddar and season with salt and freshly ground black pepper. Remove the cauliflower from the oven after about 5 minutes, stir in the bacon and jalapeños, if using, then pour over the cheese sauce. Scatter the Parmesan over the surface and return the dish to the oven for 20 to 30 minutes, or until the mixture is bubbling and brown on top. Serve with fresh greens.

Tip: substitute some of the cauliflower with broccoli to give the dish more color.

- **CALORIES** 450
- PROTEIN 20G
- FAT 39G
- FIBER 2G
- CARBS 5G

Cajun-spiced bean burgers

These tasty bean burgers offer the rich heat of the deep south.

Serves 4

7 oz celeriac (celery root), peeled and diced
3 tbsp olive oil
1 small onion, finely diced
2 garlic cloves, finely chopped
1-2 red chiles, seeded and finely diced
2 tsp Cajun spice (or see tips)
1 (14-oz) can mixed beans, rinsed and drained
Small bunch of cilantro, chopped
2 eggs, beaten
3 tbsp pine nuts, chopped
2 tsp chia seeds
1 lime, quartered
Handful of arugula leaves

Preheat the oven to 400°F. Place the celeriac in a pan of boiling water and cook for 8 to 10 minutes, or until it is tender, then drain and set aside. Heat 1 tbsp of the oil in a small frying pan, and fry the onion, garlic, chile, and Cajun spice for 2 to 3 minutes.

Transfer the mixture to a bowl, stir in the beans, celeriac, and cilantro, season well and mash energetically to bind everything together. Leave the mixture to cool slightly, then add the eggs, pine nuts, and chia seeds. Mix well to combine. With wet hands, divide the mixture into quarters and shape into patties. Put them in the fridge to chill for 30 minutes.

Drizzle 1 tbsp of the oil on a nonstick baking sheet, place the patties on it, and bake them for about 25 minutes, checking after about 15 minutes and drizzling on a bit more oil so they don't dry out. Serve on a bed of arugula leaves with a wedge of lime, and perhaps some guacamole (see page 73), and a dollop of sour cream (adds 30 calories).

Tips: you can make your own Cajun spice by combining ½ tsp each of dried oregano, paprika, cayenne pepper (or red pepper flakes), black pepper, along with ¼ tsp salt. Extra burgers can be frozen, uncooked. Bake them from frozen for 40 to 45 minutes.

- **CALORIES** 300
- PROTEIN 13G
- FAT 20G
- FIBER 1G
- CARBS 20G

Turkey burgers

Serves 6

1 lb ground turkey
  or lean pork
4 spring onions, or 1 leek,
  finely diced
4 fresh or dried apricots,
  very finely chopped
4 oz halloumi, finely diced,
  or chopped cashews
1 egg, beaten
Handful of cilantro, finely
  chopped
½ tsp red pepper flakes,
  to taste
1 tbsp olive oil

Mash the ground turkey, spring onions, apricots, halloumi, egg, cilantro, and red pepper flakes in a bowl so the flavors meld and season with salt and black pepper. Shape the mixture into 6 balls and place them on a plate. Flatten them slightly, then leave them in the fridge for half an hour to firm up. Heat the oil in a frying pan and gently fry the burgers on both sides until they are cooked through. Serve with salad (they go well with crunchy red coleslaw, see page 119) and 2 tbsp quinoa or bulgur wheat (adds 35 calories).

Tip: these are also delicious as nibbles if you make them into smaller, bite-size balls and serve them with a tasty dip such as tzatziki (see page 72).

- **CALORIES** 180
- PROTEIN 26G
- FAT 8G
- FIBER 1G
- CARBS 2G

Chinese pork meatballs

Serves 6

1 lb ground pork
2 eggs, beaten
4 spring onions, finely
  chopped
2 garlic cloves, minced,
  or 2 tsp garlic paste
½ tsp red pepper flakes
½ tsp Chinese 5 spice
1 tbsp Thai fish sauce
2 tbsp sesame oil
2 tbsp cilantro, finely
  chopped

Preheat the oven to 350°F (if baking, rather than frying; see below). Mix the ground pork, eggs, spring onions, garlic, red pepper flakes, Chinese 5 spice, fish sauce, oil, and cilantro thoroughly in a bowl, then roll the mixture into balls about the size of a plum. Either bake them on a greased baking sheet for 15 to 20 minutes or fry them gently in a pan. Serve with 1¼ lb stir-fried Swiss chard (see page 168). You could also add a portion of konjac noodles (see page 198).

- **CALORIES** 160
- PROTEIN 21G
- FAT 8G
- FIBER 1G
- CARBS 1G

Quick quiche in a dish

This no-pastry quiche was suggested by a great friend, Nicola, who sent me the recipe as a short text. It sounded too easy to be true, but it really is as simple as it is delicious.

Serves 4

4 eggs
¼ cup crème fraîche
4 oz Cheddar cheese, grated
2 spring onions, diced
4½ oz fresh spinach
½ tsp ground nutmeg

Preheat the oven to 325°F and lightly grease either an ovenproof dish or separate ramekins. With a fork whisk together the eggs and crème fraîche, then stir in the cheese, spring onions, spinach, and nutmeg with some seasoning. Pour the mixture into the dish(es) and bake for about 25 minutes (10 minutes less if using ramekins).

- **CALORIES** 280
- PROTEIN 16G
- FAT 24G
- FIBER 2G
- CARBS 1G

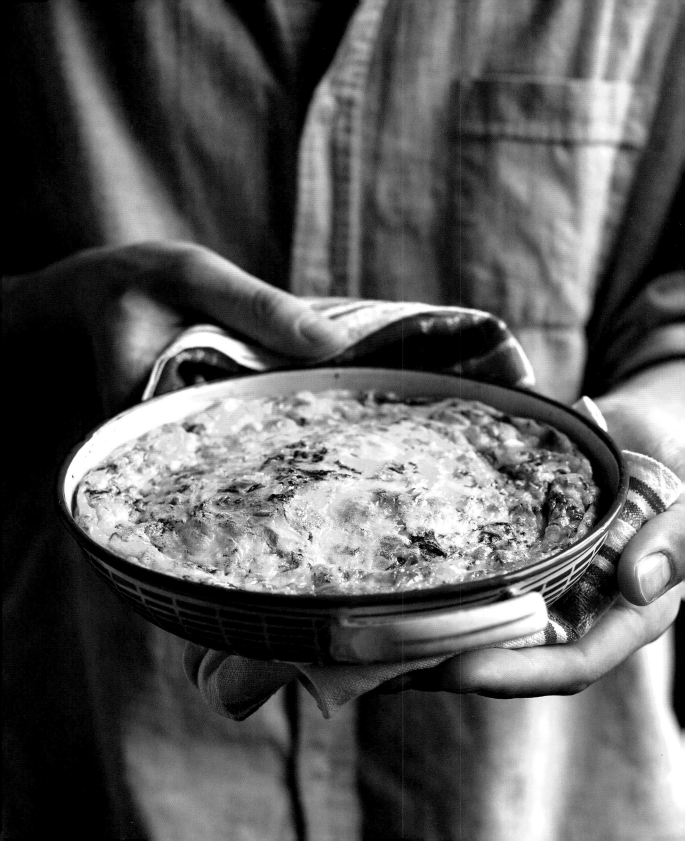

Chicken drumsticks 2 ways

1. Lightly chilied

No starchy batter or bread crumbs here. Instead, the drumsticks are lightly crusted with ground almonds, salt, pepper, and a hint of chile.

Serves 4

¼ cup ground almonds
2 oz Parmesan, grated
2 tbsp full-fat mayonnaise
2 tbsp light olive oil
1 tbsp sweet chili sauce
(from a jar, or ideally make
your own, see page 175)
8 chicken drumsticks

Preheat the oven to 350°F. Mix the almonds and Parmesan in a bowl and season well with salt and plenty of freshly ground black pepper. Mix the mayonnaise in a separate bowl with most of the oil and the chili sauce. Coat the chicken in this mixture, then roll it in the almond and Parmesan mixture. Put it in the fridge for 10 to 15 minutes to allow the crust to firm up, then place it in a greased roasting pan and drizzle the remaining oil over it. Bake it for 20 to 25 minutes, or until the juices run clear (not pink) when pierced with a sharp knife. Serve with a salad or steamed greens.

- **CALORIES** 410
- PROTEIN 31G
- FAT 30G
- FIBER 1G
- CARBS 4G

2. With a garlic crust

Serves 4

¼ cup ground almonds
2 oz Parmesan, grated
2 tbsp full-fat mayonnaise
2 tbsp light olive oil
2 tbsp Dijon mustard
2 garlic cloves, crushed
8 chicken drumsticks

Preheat the oven to 350°F. Mix the almonds and Parmesan in a bowl and season well with salt and plenty of freshly ground black pepper. Mix the mayonnaise, 1 tbsp of the oil, the mustard, and garlic in a separate bowl. Coat the chicken in this mixture, then roll it in the almond and Parmesan mixture. Put it in the fridge for 10 to 15 minutes to allow the crust to firm up, then place it in a greased roasting pan, and drizzle the remaining 1 tbsp oil over it. Bake for 20 to 25 minutes, or until the juices run clear (not pink) when pierced with a sharp knife. Serve with a salad or steamed greens.

- **CALORIES** 440
- PROTEIN 33G
- FAT 34G
- FIBER 2G
- CARBS 2G

Chicken wrapped in Parma ham

The chicken absorbs the flavors from the Parma ham which forms a delicious crust around it.

Serves 2

1 heaping tbsp full-fat cream cheese
1 garlic clove, crushed or finely chopped (or use store-bought garlic cream cheese)
2 small boneless, skinless chicken breasts
6 slices of Parma ham (or a cheaper equivalent such as prosciutto or serrano)
1 tbsp olive oil

Preheat the oven to 350°F. Mix the cream cheese and garlic and season with black pepper and a pinch of salt. Spread the mixture over the surface of the chicken breasts and wrap 2 to 3 slices of ham around each one. Drizzle the oil over the chicken, place it in an oven dish and bake for 20 to 25 minutes, or until the juices run clear (not pink) when pierced with a sharp knife. Serve with a salad or green vegetables.

- **CALORIES** 320
- PROTEIN 39G
- FAT 18G
- FIBER 0G
- CARBS 0G

Spicy tuna fish patties

This is a bit like a tuna falafel and was inspired by a recipe by Stacey on the Blood Sugar Diet website. Wonderfully quick and easy to whip together.

Serves 4

2 (6-oz) cans tuna in
  olive oil, drained
1 (14-oz) can chickpeas,
  rinsed and drained
3 spring onions, diced
½ red bell pepper, seeded
  and diced
1-2 red chiles, seeded
  and finely diced, or
  1-2 tsp chili paste or red
  pepper flakes
2 eggs
½ tsp ground cumin
2 tbsp olive oil
Juice of 2 limes
Handful of cilantro
  or parsley, chopped
  (optional)
8 small cocktail gherkins
  (around 2 oz), finely diced

Mix the tuna, chickpeas, spring onions, bell pepper, chiles, eggs, and cumin together with 1 tbsp of the oil and the juice of 1 lime in a bowl. Pulse for a few seconds with an immersion blender or a food processor, stir and pulse again for a few more seconds. This mixture should still have some texture. Then add the cilantro and gherkins and mix them in thoroughly.

Divide the mixture into 8 portions, shaping them into patties. Place them in the fridge for half an hour to firm up. Heat the remaining 1 tbsp oil in a large frying pan and fry the patties 4 at a time. When the egg has set enough for them to be turned without crumbling, flip them over. Squeeze the juice of the second lime over the patties just before serving along with tzatziki (see page 72) and a light salad or fresh greens.

Tip: if the mixture seems a bit runny, add 1 to 2 tsp chia seeds to bind it.

- **CALORIES** 310
- PROTEIN 31G
- FAT 17G
- FIBER 3G
- CARBS 11G

Indian-spiced shrimp

A deliciously light, tangy shrimp curry. Adapted from a recipe from the mother of my friend and colleague, Durgesh.

Serves 2

9-10 oz uncooked jumbo
  shrimp, shelled (or frozen
  cooked)
¼ tsp chili powder
  (to taste)
¼ tsp turmeric
1 tsp tamarind paste,
  ½ tbsp mirin, or juice
  of half a lime
1 tbsp vegetable oil
1 large onion, finely
  chopped
2 garlic cloves, crushed or
  finely chopped
1 cinnamon stick, broken
  in half
7 oz canned chopped
  tomatoes
4 oz spinach (frozen
  or fresh)

Marinate the shrimp in the chili powder, turmeric, and tamarind paste for 30 minutes. Meanwhile, heat the oil in a nonstick saucepan and sauté the onion until it starts to turn golden brown. Add the garlic and cinnamon stick. After 2 to 3 minutes, add the tomatoes and the marinade (not the shrimp). Check the seasoning and cook the sauce over medium heat until it starts to thicken. Then turn the heat to low and stir in the shrimp and spinach. Cook the shrimp until they change color if using fresh (about 10 minutes) or for about 5 minutes if they are already cooked, stirring occasionally. Serve with cauliflower rice (see page 98) or stir-fried cabbage (see page 169).

- **CALORIES** 190
- PROTEIN 24G
- FAT 7G
- FIBER 2G
- CARBS 10G

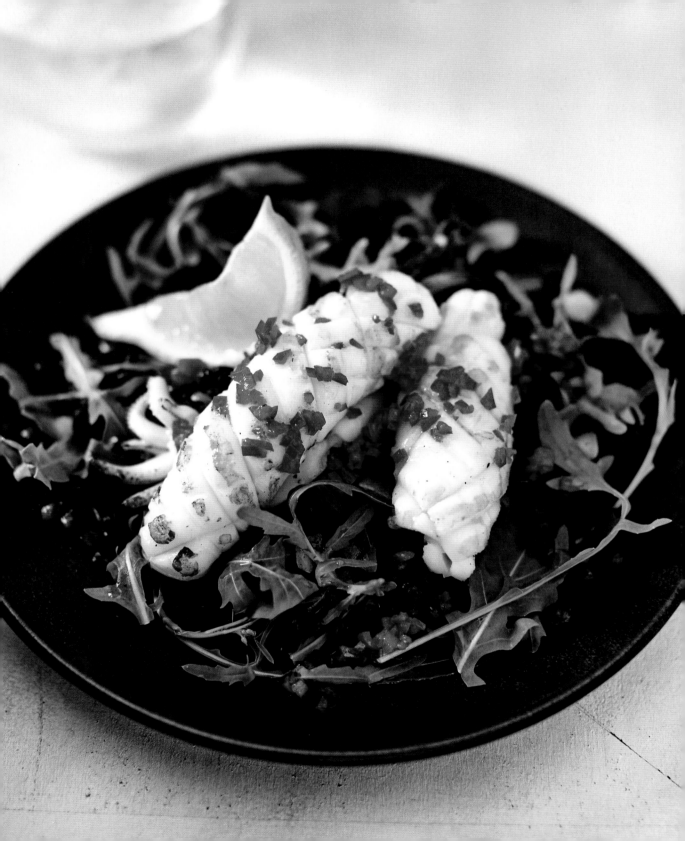

Chili squid with lentils

The chili enhances the flavors of the squid here beautifully.

Serves 4

1 small onion, diced
1 tbsp olive oil
About 9 oz store-bought
cooked Puy lentils (or cook
* from scratch)*
Juice of half a lemon
4 medium squid bodies,
* cleaned*
4 generous tsp sweet chili
* sauce (see page 175),*
* or 3 large red chiles,*
* diced and mixed with*
* 2 tbsp extra-virgin olive oil*
* and seasoned*

Prepare the lentils first. Sweat the onion in olive oil until it starts to brown. Stir in the lentils and simmer for a few minutes to heat them through. Season with salt and black pepper and the lemon juice.

Cut each squid body (tube) open, lay it flat and score the inner surface with a sharp knife in cross-hatch lines about ¼ inch apart. Season the squid and cook them on a very hot griddle with the cross-hatched side down for 1 to 2 minutes, then turn them over—they will curl up almost immediately, indicating that they are cooked.

To serve, place the lentils on the plates with the squid on top, each with a generous teaspoon of chili sauce. This dish goes well with an arugula salad, drizzled with olive oil and lemon juice.

Tip: home-cooked Puy lentils taste even better, with a slightly stronger peppery flavor.

- **CALORIES** 160
- PROTEIN 18G
- FAT 5G
- FIBER 3G
- CARBS 13G

Salmon 3 ways

1. With lemon and dill nut crust on roasted vegetables

Serves 4

3 bell peppers, preferably
  red and yellow, chopped
  into large pieces
2 zucchini, coarsely sliced
2 red onions, cut into
  wedges
Drizzle of olive oil
1 egg
Grated zest of 1 lemon
Handful of dill, minced
1 tbsp crushed walnuts
2 tbsp ground almonds
4 salmon fillets

Preheat the oven to 350°F. Put the bell peppers, zucchini, and onions in a baking dish or pan, season them and drizzle with the oil. Start baking them while you prepare the fish. Beat the egg in a bowl and add the lemon zest, dill, walnuts, and almonds and mix well. Season with a pinch of salt and plenty of black pepper.

Remove the vegetables from the oven after 10 minutes and place the salmon on top, leaving a gap between each fillet. Spoon the nut mixture evenly over each fillet and return them to the oven for another 15 to 20 minutes (be careful not to overcook them as they will dry out).

- **CALORIES** 370
- PROTEIN 28G
- FAT 23G
- FIBER 4G
- CARBS 14G

2. With coconut and chile

A fabulous and easy Indian recipe by our good friends, Drs. Rajsingh and Rai.

Serves 1

1 salmon fillet
1 tsp lemon juice
1 tsp light olive oil
1 small onion, diced
¾ inch fresh ginger, grated
2 garlic cloves, minced
1-2 green chiles, seeded
  and diced (to taste)
Handful of cilantro,
  coarsely chopped
1 tbsp grated fresh coconut,
  or ½ tbsp desiccated
  coconut

Preheat the oven to 350°F. Season the fish, drizzle with lemon juice, and leave it to marinate for 30 to 60 minutes. Heat the oil in a small frying pan and sauté the onion until it is soft, about 5 minutes. Add the ginger, garlic, chiles, and cilantro and continue to cook gently on medium heat for 2 to 3 minutes before adding the coconut and salt to taste. Stir for another minute, then remove the pan from the heat. Place the fish in a baking pan and spread the mixture over it. Bake for about 20 minutes. Serve with steamed green vegetables such as snow peas or haricots verts.

Tip: fresh grated coconut can be kept in the freezer.

- **CALORIES** 300
- PROTEIN 22G
- FAT 20G
- FIBER 3G
- CARBS 7G

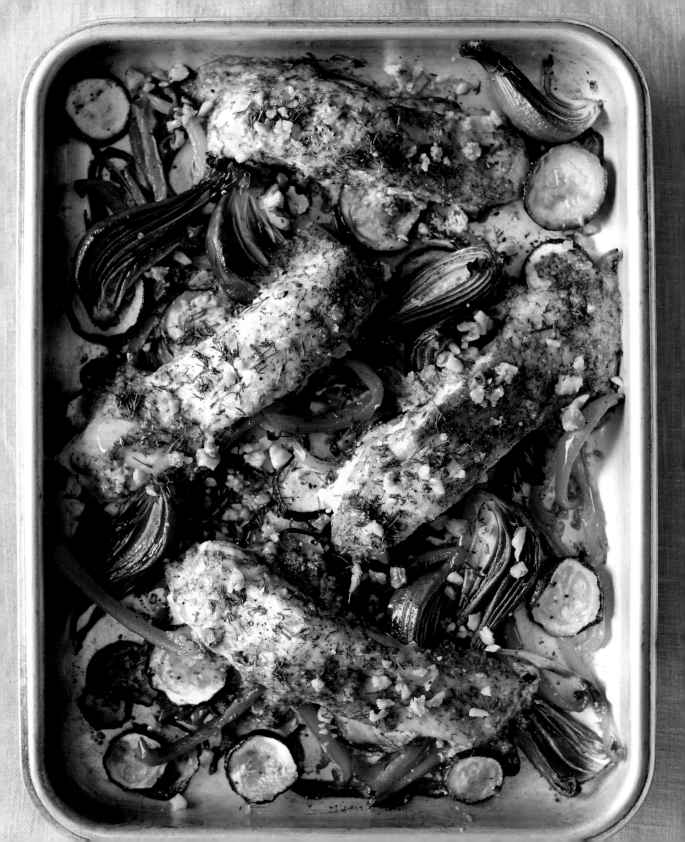

3. With ginger

This is an old favorite of ours. Purists may prefer to swap the ginger in syrup for fresh ginger, but the tiny amount of extra sugar eaten with the meal is insignificant.

Serves 6

6 medium salmon fillets
2 tbsp Thai fish sauce
3 spring onions, sliced
   lengthwise
2 red bell peppers, seeded
   and cut into strips
Juice of 1 medium orange
1 piece of ginger in syrup,
   drained and finely diced
1 red chile, seeded and
   finely chopped
½ tbsp olive oil
Handful of cilantro or
   parsley, chopped

Preheat the oven to 350°F. Place the salmon in a shallow baking dish to marinate in the fish sauce for 10 to 20 minutes. Scatter the spring onions and red pepper strips around the salmon, then pour over the orange juice. Sprinkle the ginger and chile on top. Drizzle with the oil and season well. Bake the salmon for about 20 minutes. Sprinkle with the cilantro and serve with green vegetables such as kale or spring greens.

- **CALORIES 210**
- PROTEIN 21G
- FAT 11G
- FIBER 1G
- CARBS 5G

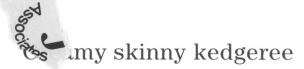

my skinny kedgeree

Serves 2

2 eggs
⅔ cup low-fat milk
2 bay leaves
6 oz smoked white fish,
 such as haddock
½ large cauliflower, grated
2 small onions, one diced,
 one cut finely into rings
2 tbsp coconut oil, or 3 tbsp
 butter
2 tsp medium curry powder
 (1 tsp if using hot variety)
1½ oz (1 heaping tbsp)
 cooked peas (optional)
Squeeze of lemon (to taste)
Handful of parsley, chopped

Boil the eggs for 6 to 7 minutes, then plunge them into cold water to cool them before peeling and cutting them in half. Meanwhile, pour the milk into a small saucepan with a lid. Add the bay leaves and fish (this can be cut up if necessary so that it lies flat) and simmer for 10 minutes. Remove the fish to a plate, keeping the milk in the pan. Allow the fish to cool a bit before removing the skin and flaking the flesh. Add the cauliflower to the milk and simmer for 5 to 7 minutes. Drain the milk into a bowl and put the cauliflower aside.

In a large frying pan, gently cook the diced onion in 1 tbsp of the oil for 5 minutes. Stir in the curry powder and cook gently for another 2 to 3 minutes. Then fold in the cauliflower, flaked fish, and peas, if using, with enough of the infused milk to loosen the mixture. Simmer for a few minutes. Pour in extra milk if it seems to be drying out.

While the cauliflower cooks, in a separate pan, fry the onion rings in the remaining 1 tbsp oil until they are golden brown and slightly crispy. Add a squeeze of lemon to the kedgeree and serve it with the eggs on top, the onion rings, and parsley scattered over, along with a grinding of black pepper.

- **CALORIES** 390
- PROTEIN 30G
- FAT 24G
- FIBER 3G
- CARBS 12G

Rice swaps

Unfortunately, white rice is high in starch and rapidly leads to a spike in blood sugar in most people. Brown rice is better, but should still be eaten only occasionally. You can reduce the impact of eating brown rice on your blood sugar levels by adding 1 to 2 teaspoons of oil to the boiling water during cooking and then leaving it in the fridge for 12 hours (1 ounce or 2 tablespoons plus 1 teaspoon brown rice = 130 calories). Cooking and then cooling rice converts the carbohydrate in it into "resistant" starch, a form which is more like fiber, and therefore has a lower GI. As brown rice takes longer to cook than white rice, we recommend keeping prepared portions in the freezer. Not only will it be ready almost instantly when needed, but some of it will have become resistant starch in the process. Win win.

Cauliflower rice

This is a surprisingly good, low-carb replacement for rice. High in fiber and nutrients, cauliflower contains astonishingly few calories and has a very low GI. It has become so popular that supermarkets are selling it in their freezer section. If you are preparing your own, first grate your cauliflower (or blitz it in a food processor). Then there are various ways of cooking it (1 medium cauliflower makes 4 servings of 30 calories each):

BAKED: mix it with 1 teaspoon olive oil in a bowl then bake it in a medium oven for about 10 minutes—it will need occasional shaking and turning (adds 30 calories per portion).

MICROWAVED: in a covered bowl for a minute or two until it's al dente and still slightly chewy.

STEAMED: for 5 to 7 minutes.

FRIED: simply fry it in 1 tablespoon olive oil for 7 to 8 minutes until it's al dente (adds 30 calories per portion).

Konjac rice

This is sold as "low-carb rice" in precooked packages. It is made of konjac glucomannan, a natural soluble fiber, and, like konjac noodle products, is very low in starchy carbohydrates and gluten-free. Konjac rice has a slightly rubbery texture and is best rinsed before use. It has no particular flavor of its own and works well when mixed with strong flavors such as in stir-fries, Asian salads, or soups.

Quinoa

This has become an incredibly popular replacement for grains. If, like me, you are struggling with the pronunciation—it is pronounced "keen-wah." Like buckwheat, it is a pseudo-cereal and has a slightly nutty taste and chewy texture. Quinoa has significantly higher levels of protein, nutrients, and fiber than rice and much less impact on blood sugars. But it is starchy, like brown rice, so eat it in moderation, 1 to 2 tablespoons per serving. We particularly recommend the darker brown and red varieties, as these have a higher fiber content and more taste. It is very easy to cook.

Serves 2

⅓ cup quinoa
1 cup plus 2 tbsp chicken
  or vegetable stock

In a small saucepan, cover the quinoa with about ¼ to ¾ inch of stock and bring it to a boil. Put the lid on and turn down the heat to a simmer for 10 minutes, or until the water is absorbed. Then turn off the heat and let it steam with the lid on for another 10 minutes.

- CALORIES 120
- PROTEIN 6G
- FAT 2G
- FIBER 2G
- CARBS 22G

Bulgur wheat

Although bulgur wheat is not as high in protein or as low-carb as quinoa, it does have a fairly high fiber content.

Serves 2

⅔ cup bulgur wheat
¾-1 cup chicken or
  vegetable stock

In a small saucepan, cover the bulgur with about ¼-¾ inch of stock and bring it to a boil. Put the lid on and turn down the heat to a simmer for 10 minutes. Then turn off the heat and let it steam with the lid on for another 10 minutes.

- CALORIES 140
- PROTEIN 4G
- FAT 1G
- FIBER 3G
- CARBS 31G

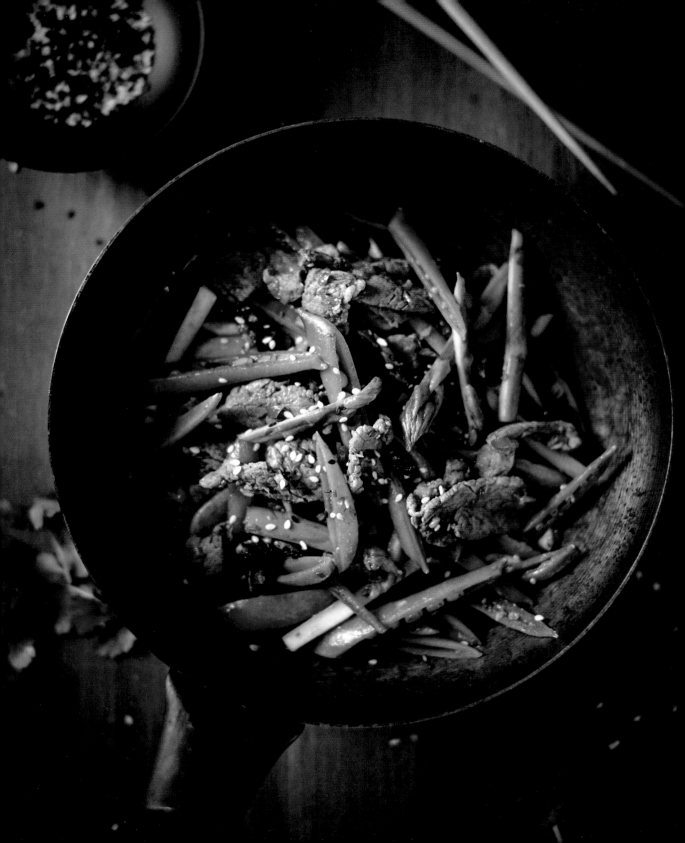

Beef stir-fry with asparagus and sesame seeds

We include asparagus here mainly because it tastes so delicious and complements the flavors. However, it also happens to contain plenty of inulin, which acts as a prebiotic, boosting the beneficial bacteria in the gut, and thereby helping to keep weight off and your blood sugars down.

Serves 2

1 tbsp mirin or sherry
2 tbsp soy sauce
¾ inch fresh ginger, grated
1 garlic clove, minced
1 red chile, seeded and finely diced, or 1 tsp red pepper flakes
7 oz beef fillet, thinly sliced
7 oz canned black beans
1 tbsp coconut or rapeseed oil
5 oz asparagus, cut into 1½ inch batons (if thick, slice the stalks length-wise too)
4 oz snow peas or sugar snap peas, chopped into thin sticks (optional)
1 tsp sesame oil (optional)
2 tsp sesame seeds
Handful of cilantro leaves, torn

Mix the mirin, ½ tbsp of the soy sauce, the ginger, garlic, and chile in a bowl and marinate the beef fillet in it for 30 minutes. In a separate small bowl, marinate the beans in ½ tbsp of the soy sauce. Place a wok over high heat, add the coconut oil, and then the beef mixture. Stir-fry for about 2 minutes, or until the meat is browned all over. Add the asparagus, snow peas, if using, beans and sesame oil and reduce the heat. Then stir in 2 tbsp of hot water and the remaining 1 tbsp soy sauce and stir-fry gently for another minute or two, until the vegetables are just tender. Season with freshly ground black pepper and sprinkle with the sesame seeds and cilantro leaves. Serve with cauliflower rice (see page 98).

- **CALORIES** 250
- PROTEIN 27G
- FAT 13G
- FIBER 3G
- CARBS 5G

Chickpeas 2 ways

Chickpeas, one of the legumes recommended as part of a healthy Mediterranean-style diet, are quite high in protein, nutrients, and fiber. They are also fairly high in carbohydrate, but when combined with vegetables and healthy oils the carbs are released relatively slowly, providing energy without significantly spiking blood sugars.

1. With Indian-spiced stir-fried greens

A delicious, quick meal that also works well as a side dish.

Serves 2

1 tbsp coconut or
  rapeseed oil
1 tsp mustard seeds
1 large onion, diced
  fairly small
5-6 curry leaves
2 green chiles, seeded
  and diced, or 2 tsp red
  pepper flakes (to taste)
½ tsp turmeric
7 oz canned white lentils
7 oz canned chickpeas
1 lb green cabbage,
  thinly sliced
1 tsp garam masala

Heat the oil in a large nonstick, wok-style pan. Add the mustard seeds and then the onion, curry leaves, and chiles. Sauté for 3 to 4 minutes on low heat. Stir in the turmeric, lentils, chickpeas, and cabbage. Season with salt, and cook on high heat for 5 to 7 minutes, stirring constantly. Finally, mix in the garam masala and season to taste.

Tip: you can use dried chickpeas and lentils and boil them (separately) until they are al dente. Use about 4 oz of each, cooked and drained.

- **CALORIES** 390
- PROTEIN 22G
- FAT 13G
- FIBER 18G
- CARBS 51G

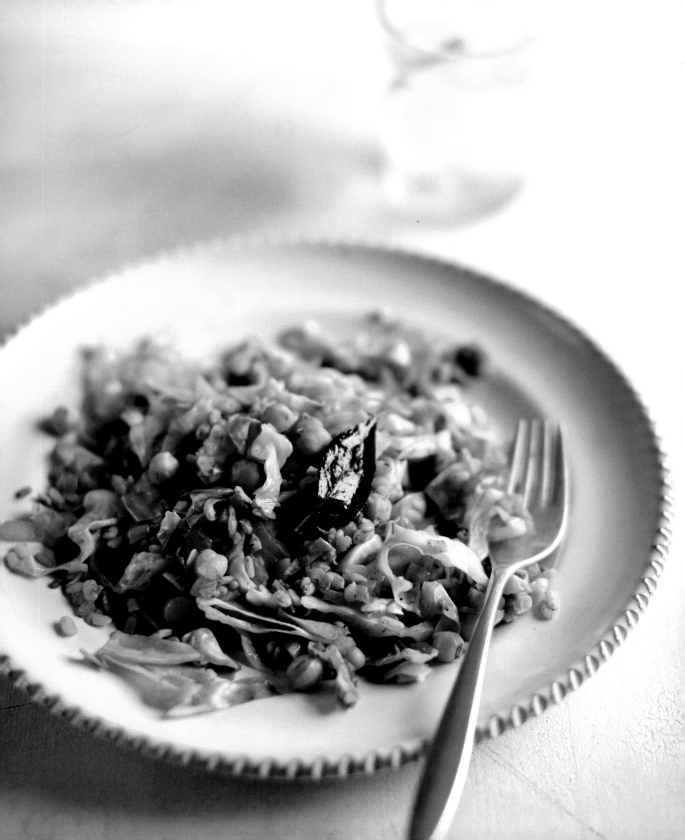

2. Chickpea chili

A rich, vegetarian dish, super-easy to make.

Serves 2

2 tbsp olive oil
1 medium onion, diced
1 tsp ground cumin
½ tsp dried oregano
1 carrot, diced
1 red bell pepper, seeded
  and diced
2 celery stalks, diced
4 oz mushrooms, chopped
1 garlic clove, diced or
  crushed
1 green chile, seeded and
  diced (more if you like it
  hot), or 1 tsp chili paste or
  red pepper flakes)
1 (14-oz) can chopped
  tomatoes
½ tbsp balsamic vinegar
1 (14-oz) can chickpeas
7 oz canned black beans or
  kidney beans
Handful of cilantro leaves,
  chopped

Heat the oil in a large saucepan and gently cook the onion for 5 minutes. Add the cumin and oregano, then the carrot, bell pepper, celery, and mushrooms, and cook for another 10 minutes. Stir in the garlic, chile, tomatoes, vinegar, chickpeas, and beans, and simmer vigorously until the sauce has begun to reduce, about 10 minutes. Season to taste and serve with a scattering of cilantro and a spoonful of raita (see page 72).

Tips: this recipe works well with other types of beans. You could also include diced eggplant or zucchini. It's very flexible.

- CALORIES 270
- PROTEIN 13G
- FAT 9G
- FIBER 10G
- CARBS 36G

Stir-fried cabbage with peppered mackerel

So simple and delicious. I could live on this.

Serves 2

1 tbsp olive oil
1 small onion, sliced
1 garlic clove, chopped
About ¾ lb cabbage or
  spring greens, finely sliced
2 peppered smoked
  mackerel fillets

Heat the oil in a large frying pan and gently cook the onion and garlic for 5 minutes, or until they have softened. Add the cabbage and some seasoning and stir-fry for 2 to 3 minutes. Remove the skin from the mackerel and flake the flesh into the pan for the last minute of cooking.

Tip: you can use other smoked fish for this recipe but you may need to add extra pepper and perhaps a scattering of chile to enhance the flavors.

- CALORIES 280
- PROTEIN 13G
- FAT 22G
- FIBER 4G
- CARBS 9G

Chicken biriani with cauli rice

Cauliflower rice works brilliantly with chicken biriani and dramatically reduces the amount of starchy carbohydrates involved.

Serves 4

3 tbsp coconut oil, or
  ¼ cup butter
1 large cauliflower, grated
2 tbsp sliced almonds
2 large onions, 1 sliced
  finely into rings, 1 diced
2 garlic cloves, minced
¾ inch fresh ginger, grated
Seeds from 3 cardamom
  pods
1 cinnamon stick, broken
  in half
1 tsp turmeric
4 medium boneless,
  skinless chicken
  breasts, cut into ¾-inch
  chunks
2-3 tbsp medium curry
  paste
About ⅔ cup raisins
¼-½ cup chicken stock
Generous handful of
  cilantro, chopped

Preheat the oven to 350°F. Drizzle 1 tbsp of the oil over the cauliflower, spread it out on a baking sheet and bake for 10 minutes, shaking the tray and turning the cauliflower a few times during cooking.

Meanwhile, toast the almonds in a dry nonstick frying pan for a few minutes, until they start to turn golden brown, then set them aside. Using the same pan, gently fry the onion rings in 1 tbsp of the oil until they are golden brown, then set them aside, too.

In another large nonstick saucepan, heat the remaining 1 tbsp oil and fry the diced onions, garlic, ginger, and spices for 5 to 10 minutes, or until the onions are golden brown. Transfer this mixture to a bowl and use the same pan to fry the chicken with the curry paste in the remaining 1 tbsp oil. Once the chicken is cooked—this should take 5 to 10 minutes—stir in the cauliflower rice along with the raisins, stock, and spicy onion mix. Cover the pan and simmer for 4 to 5 minutes, then stir through half the cilantro. Top the biriani with the fried onion rings, the rest of the cilantro, and the toasted almonds. Serve with raita (see page 72) and some steamed greens.

- **CALORIES** 390
- PROTEIN 32G
- FAT 17G
- FIBER 4G
- CARBS 29G

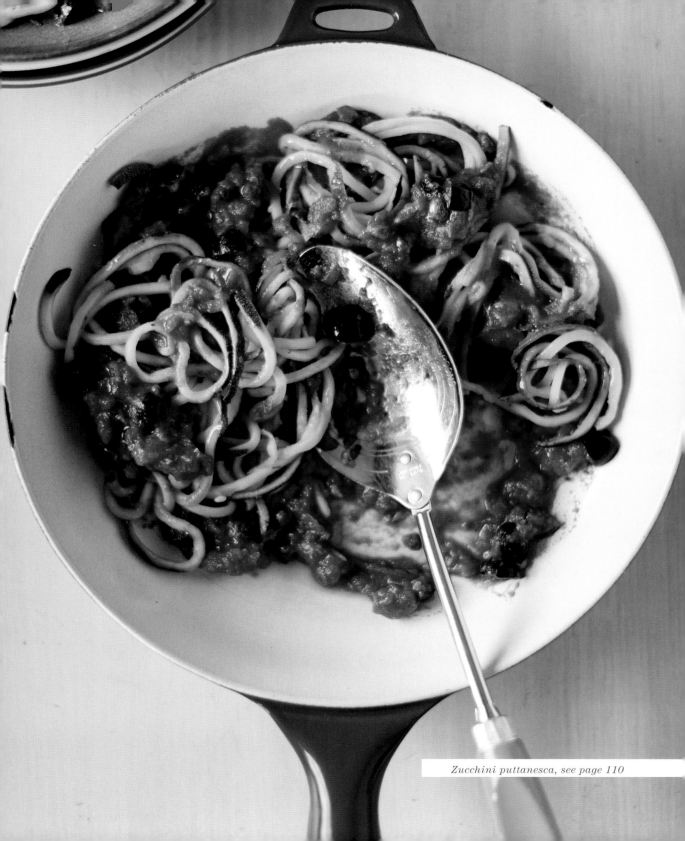

Zucchini puttanesca, see page 110

Guilt-free spaghetti

Despite being part of the Mediterranean diet, pasta is a high-GI, starchy food that is broken down rapidly into sugars. And unfortunately brown pasta is not much better.

For those of us trying to find alternatives to pasta, a spiralizer, which looks a bit like a giant serrated pencil sharpener and shreds chunks of vegetables into wonderful strands of "vegetti," has become one of the must-have pieces of kitchen equipment. We have a fairly low-tech kitchen—most of the gadgets we do have lurk somewhere toward the back of the kitchen drawers. But the spiralizer is still right up there at the front. It works best on firm vegetables like carrots, zucchini, butternut squash, celeriac (and if this all sounds too much like hard work, the good news is that you can now buy prepared spiralized vegetables at most supermarkets).

Other spaghetti alternatives:
Konjac-based low-carb noodles (see page 198)
Finely sliced cabbage, steamed or boiled
Green beans, cut lengthwise (available in some supermarkets, frozen are fine)

Zucchini noodles 6 ways

1. With pesto, goat cheese, and peas

Serves 2

¾ cup frozen peas
1 tbsp pine nuts
3 tbsp pesto sauce (either homemade, see pg 177; or from a jar)
1 large zucchini (about 7 oz), spiralized
2 oz goat cheese

Boil the peas for 4 to 5 minutes, then drain them and set them aside. In a dry nonstick frying pan, toast the pine nuts until they turn golden at the edges (1 to 2 minutes) and set them aside. Steam, microwave, or boil the zucchini for about 2 minutes, or until it is al dente. In a bowl, mix the zucchini noodles, peas, and pesto, then crumble in the goat cheese and stir gently. Sprinkle the pine nuts on top and serve.

- **CALORIES** 420
- PROTEIN 22G
- FAT 31G
- FIBER 6G
- CARBS 12G

2. With bacon and beans

Serves 2

4 oz diced bacon, lardons,
  or pancetta
1 tbsp olive oil
1 garlic clove, crushed
5 oz canned fava beans
  or other beans, such
  as cannellini or haricots
  verts, rinsed and drained
2 heaping tbsp crème
  fraîche
1 large zucchini (about
  7 oz), spiralized
Small handful of parsley,
  chopped
1 tbsp grated Parmesan

Gently fry the bacon in the oil in a medium frying pan until it is slightly browned, then turn down the heat and add the garlic and the beans. Sauté for a few more minutes then remove the pan from the heat and allow the mixture to cool for a few minutes before stirring in the crème fraîche.

Steam, microwave, or boil the zucchini noodles for 2 to 3 minutes, or until they are al dente. Mix all the cooked ingredients in a bowl, then add the parsley, and scatter with the Parmesan.

Tip: we use canned beans but you can use frozen or fresh (which will need cooking first).

- CALORIES 270
- PROTEIN 16G
- FAT 20G
- FIBER 5G
- CARBS 7G

---

3. With seafood

This tastes of holidays beside the sea—it's been my favorite pasta dish since I was a teenager. And now it's got even better.

Serves 2

1 tbsp olive oil
2 garlic cloves, finely sliced
Pinch of red pepper flakes
¾ lb frozen mixed seafood
1 oz samphire or green
  beans, lightly chopped
Zest of half a lemon
1 large zucchini (about
  7 oz), spiralized
1 tbsp pine nuts, toasted
Handful of basil leaves,
  torn, or 1 tsp dried

Heat the oil in a medium frying pan and gently cook the garlic with the red pepper flakes for a few minutes until it has softened. Add the seafood and cook gently for another 3 minutes. Then add the samphire and cook for 2 to 3 minutes more. Give the pan a good shake to distribute the ingredients evenly and then sprinkle on the lemon zest.

Steam, microwave, or boil the zucchini noodles for 2 to 3 minutes, or until they are al dente. Season and serve with the seafood piled on top, and the pine nuts and basil sprinkled on top.

Tip: Samphire is a sea vegetable. Use green beans if you can't find it.

- CALORIES 230
- PROTEIN 29G
- FAT 10G
- FIBER 1G
- CARBS 8G

4. With tomato meatballs

A classic dish, now with a healthy spiralized twist.

Serves 2

7 oz ground beef (or any
  other ground meat)
¼ cup grated Parmesan
1 onion, finely diced
1 egg, beaten
½ tbsp Worcestershire
  sauce (or other flavoring
  depending on the meat)
Small handful of parsley,
  finely chopped
2 tbsp olive oil
Pinch of dried oregano or
  thyme
1 garlic clove, crushed
½ tsp red pepper flakes
1 (14 oz) can tomatoes
1 large zucchini (about
  7 oz), spiralized

In a bowl, mix the ground beef, half the Parmesan, half the onion, the egg, Worcestershire sauce, and parsley and season well. With your hands, work at the mixture for a few minutes, squidging the ingredients together and mopping up the egg. Divide the mixture into plum-size balls and put them in the fridge to firm up for 20 minutes before frying.

To make the tomato sauce, in a medium saucepan, gently cook the rest of the onion in 1 tbsp of the oil for 5 minutes, then stir in the oregano, garlic, and red pepper flakes. After 2 more minutes, add the tomatoes. Simmer, uncovered, for about 20 minutes, until the sauce has thickened and reduced.

Fry the meatballs in a separate frying pan in the remaining 1 tbsp oil for about 5 minutes, then add them to the simmering tomato sauce, to finish cooking.

Steam, microwave, or boil the zucchini noodles for 2 to 3 minutes, or until it is al dente. Serve it with the tomato meatballs on top, scattered with the remaining Parmesan.

- **CALORIES** 390
- PROTEIN 39G
- FAT 21G
- FIBER 3G
- CARBS 14G

5. Carbonara

Serves 2

¼ cup grated Parmesan
2 large egg yolks
4 tbsp heavy cream
2 oz turkey bacon, diced
1 tbsp olive oil
1 garlic clove, crushed
1 large zucchini (about
  7 oz), spiralized

Put half the cheese into a bowl, add the egg yolks and heavy cream, season with black pepper and whisk everything together.

In a medium saucepan, fry the bacon in the oil for 4 to 5 minutes, then add the garlic and zucchini noodles and cook for another few minutes. Stir in the sauce, ensuring that everything is well coated, and serve with the remaining Parmesan sprinkled on top.

- **CALORIES** 490
- PROTEIN 15G
- FAT 47G
- FIBER 1G
- CARBS 3G

---

6. Puttanesca

Full of healthy Mediterranean ingredients, including anchovies, which bring a delicate salty taste. Excellent for reluctant fish eaters.

Serves 2

4 anchovies from a jar or
  can, drained and chopped
1 garlic clove, crushed
¼-½ tsp red pepper flakes
  or fresh chile, seeded
  and finely diced
2 tbsp olive oil
7 oz canned tomatoes
2 tbsp capers, rinsed
2 oz pitted black olives,
  sliced
1 tsp dried oregano
1 large zucchini (about
  7 oz), spiralized

Over a gentle heat, fry the anchovies, garlic, and red pepper flakes in the oil for 2 to 3 minutes. Press the anchovies against the pan with a wooden spoon to form a paste. Then add the tomatoes, capers, and olives and cook gently for 20 to 30 minutes without a lid. About 5 minutes before the sauce is ready, steam, microwave, or boil the zucchini noodles for 2 to 3 minutes, so that they are still slightly al dente. Serve the sauce on top of the zucchini noodles along with a light salad.

- **CALORIES** 160
- PROTEIN 4G
- FAT 15G
- FIBER 2G
- CARBS 4G

Shrimp and tuna fried rice

This delicious seafood fried rice can be made almost entirely from items that you are likely to have on hand.

Serves 2

½ tbsp coconut or
  rapeseed oil
1 onion, chopped
½ tsp red pepper flakes or
  fresh chile, seeded and
  finely diced (to taste)
1 garlic clove, chopped
¼ inch fresh ginger,
  chopped
1 red bell pepper, seeded
  and chopped
7 oz cauliflower rice (see
  page 98)
4 oz shrimp (fresh or
  frozen and thawed)
4 oz canned tuna
1 tbsp Thai fish sauce
7 oz Chinese vegetables
  or cabbage, diced
2 eggs, beaten
Handful of cilantro, torn

Heat the oil in a wok and fry the onion, red pepper flakes, garlic, and ginger for 1 to 2 minutes before adding the bell pepper and, after 4 to 5 minutes, the cauliflower rice. After a couple more minutes, stir in the shrimp, tuna, fish sauce, and the Chinese vegetables. (If using fresh shrimp, cook them until they are pink before adding the other ingredients.) Continue to fry gently for another few minutes. Finally, clear a hollow in the center of the wok in which to scramble the eggs. Stir them through, season, and garnish the dish with the cilantro.

- CALORIES 290
- PROTEIN 34G
- FAT 12G
- FIBER 5G
- CARBS 13G

High-protein salads

These salads are all potentially meals in themselves. You don't need to stick to the exact ingredients—go with what you have to hand or what is in season.

Watercress, orange, and sardine salad

A wonderful combination of flavors and textures—even better with fresh sardines.

Serves 2

2 oranges (including the zest of one)
1 tbsp olive oil
Juice of half a lemon
4 oz watercress
½ red onion, thinly sliced
Handful of tarragon or cilantro leaves, torn
4 oz can sardines in oil, drained (or fresh sardines if available, see tip)
1 tbsp pumpkin seeds

In a bowl, make a dressing by whisking together the orange zest, oil, and lemon juice with some salt and pepper. Peel both oranges, removing as much pith as possible, and cut them into slices. Arrange the watercress, onion, and tarragon leaves in a bowl, add the slices of orange and then the sardines. Drizzle with the dressing and sprinkle with pumpkin seeds.

Tip: if you have a good fishmonger, it is well worth using fresh sardines (allow 2 per person). Buy them scaled and gutted, with heads and gills removed. Rub them with olive oil, generous amounts of salt and ground pepper, and cook them on a grill or griddle pan for about 5 minutes, turning once. They are cooked if the flesh in the thickest part of the fish pulls away easily.

- **CALORIES** 320
- PROTEIN 19G
- FAT 19G
- FIBER 4G
- CARBS 19G

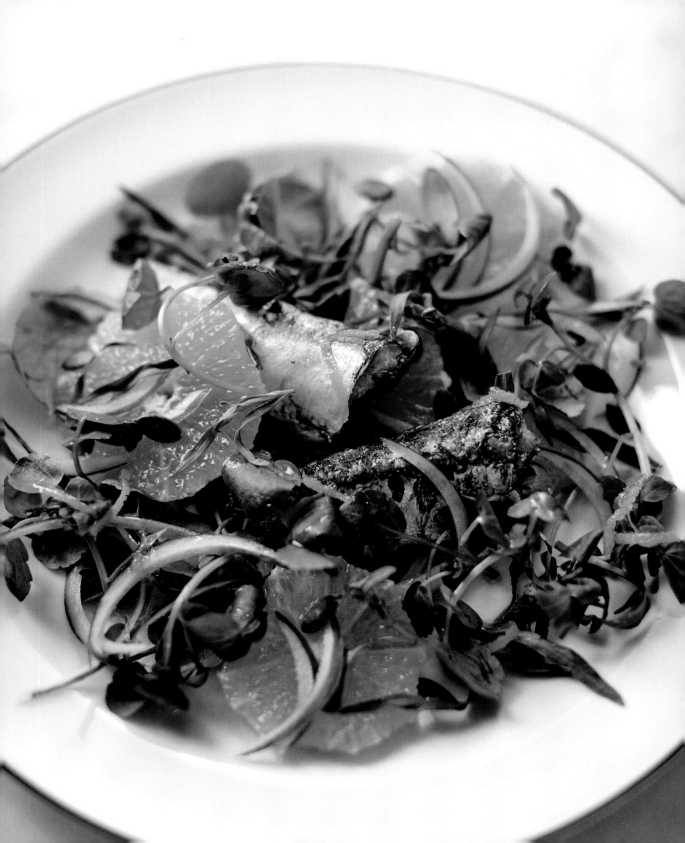

Endive 2 ways

Endive is a wonderful vegetable, providing the nutritional benefits that often come with bitter foods. Sadly, it is too sharp a flavor for modern tastes. It also has high levels of inulin, a form of fiber which encourages the growth of healthy bacteria in your gut. All good to keep the sugars down.

1. With anchovy mayo

The slight bitterness of endive is counteracted by the creamy mayonnaise here. A delicious and interesting combination.

Serves 2

1 tbsp full-fat mayonnaise
1 tbsp extra-virgin olive oil
1 tbsp lime juice
1 level tbsp minced
 rosemary leaves
3 anchovy fillets from a jar
 or can, finely diced
2 heads endive
Large handful of arugula or
 baby lettuce leaves
½ red bell pepper, seeded
 and diced (optional)

Mix the mayonnaise, oil, and lime well, then add the rosemary and anchovies and blitz with an immersion blender or mix energetically with a spoon to infuse the flavors. Discard the outer leaves of the endive and separate the rest from the stalk. Arrange the leaves on a serving plate with the arugula and the bell pepper, if using. Drizzle with the anchovy dressing and season generously with freshly ground black pepper.

- **CALORIES** 170
- PROTEIN 3G
- FAT 16G
- FIBER 2G
- CARBS 6G

2. With pear, hazelnut, and goat cheese

Serves 2

2 tbsp olive oil
1 tbsp cider vinegar
2 heads endive
1 pear, cored and sliced
2 oz goat cheese, diced
Handful of arugula leaves
2 tbsp chopped hazelnuts,
 toasted

In a bowl, make a dressing by whisking together the oil and vinegar with some salt and pepper. Discard the outer leaves of the endive and separate the rest from the stalk. Arrange the leaves on 2 plates, with the pear slices and cheese on top. Drizzle with the dressing and scatter the arugula leaves and nuts on top.

- **CALORIES** 310
- PROTEIN 9G
- FAT 26G
- FIBER 4G
- CARBS 12G

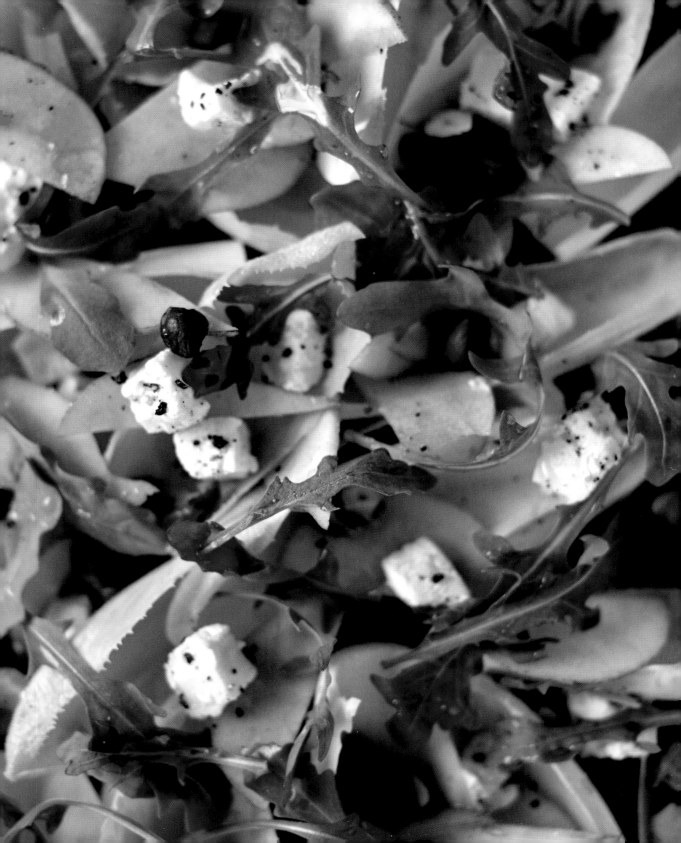

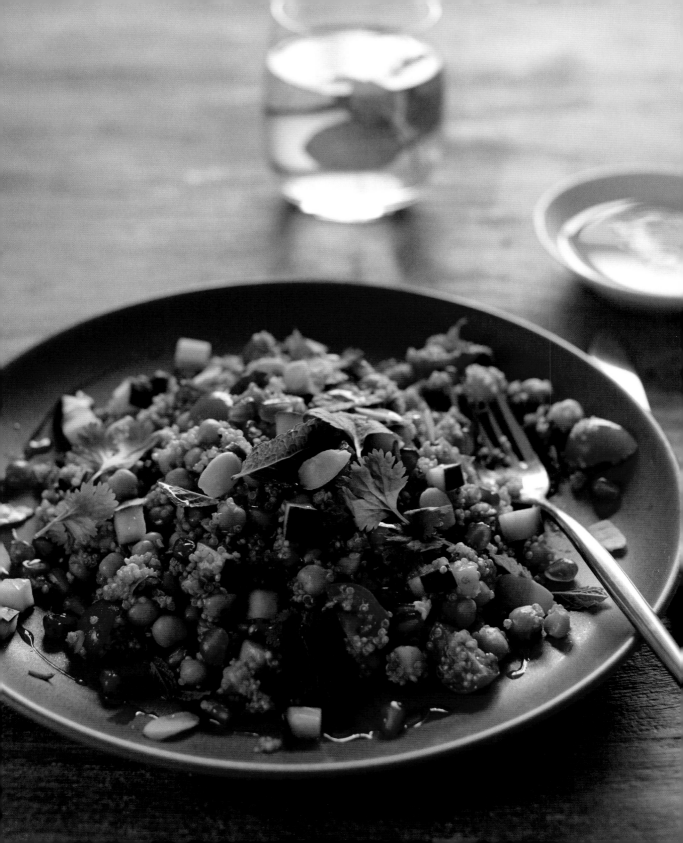

Moroccan spiced chickpea salad

We use quinoa here instead of couscous as it is higher in protein and fiber and significantly lower in starchy carbohydrates.

Serves 4

1 cup quinoa (mixture of dark and pale if available)
1½ cups vegetable stock
1 (14 oz) can chickpeas, rinsed and drained
1 tbsp olive oil
Juice of 1 lemon
1 tsp ras el hanout, harissa paste, or paprika
8 cherry tomatoes, halved
¼ cucumber, seeded and diced
4 spring onions, finely chopped
½ cup pomegranate seeds or raisins
Handful of mint or cilantro leaves, torn
2 tbsp sliced almonds, toasted

Place the quinoa in a saucepan with the stock, bring it to a boil, then reduce the heat and simmer for 10 to 15 minutes, or until all the stock has been absorbed. Remove from the heat, cover, and let stand for 5 more minutes.

Put the chickpeas into a wide bowl and add the oil, lemon, and ras el hanout. Mix well to coat the chickpeas. Add the quinoa and tomatoes, cucumber, spring onions, pomegranate seeds, mint, and almonds to the chickpeas and gently toss them together. Season with salt and freshly ground black pepper.

Tip: seed the cucumber by cutting it in half lengthwise and scooping out the watery seeds with a teaspoon.

- **CALORIES** 400
- PROTEIN 15G
- FAT 14G
- FIBER 8G
- CARBS 60G

Lentil, carrot, and avocado salad

A perfect combination of Mediterranean goodness.

Serves 2

11 oz carrots, cut into
  batons (short sticks)
1 tbsp olive oil
1 tsp cumin seeds
2 handfuls of mâche
  leaves
4 oz canned Puy lentils,
  rinsed and drained
1 avocado, sliced
2 tsp sesame seeds
1 tbsp raisins
Juice of half a lemon, or
  1 tbsp cider vinegar

Preheat the oven to 400°F. Toss the carrots in the oil and cumin seeds in a baking pan and roast for 20 minutes. Leave the carrots to cool for a few minutes. Place the lettuce in a bowl with the lentils and avocado. Add the carrots and sprinkle with the sesame seeds and raisins, followed by a generous squeeze of lemon and some salt and black pepper.

Tip: to convert this salad into a more substantial meal, you could add a handful of nuts and/or crumbled feta and adjust the calories accordingly.

- **CALORIES** 330
- PROTEIN 8G
- FAT 20G
- FIBER 8G
- CARBS 31G

Shrimp, pea, and spring onion salad

A lovely light summery salad.

Serves 2

4 oz frozen peas
Zest and juice of half
  a lemon
½ cup crème fraîche
Handful of chives, snipped
2 Boston lettuce heads,
  chopped
7 oz cooked shrimp
3 spring onions, finely
  sliced

Cook the peas in a pan of boiling water for 5 minutes. Drain them, rinse under cold water, and set them aside. Whisk the lemon zest and juice with the crème fraîche, season with salt and pepper, and stir in the chives. Place the lettuce in a bowl, add the shrimp, peas, and spring onions and toss everything in the chive dressing.

- **CALORIES** 300
- PROTEIN 20G
- FAT 21G
- FIBER 3G
- CARBS 8G

Roasted beet and fig salad

The tangy beet is a perfect foil for the sweet figs and salty feta.

Serves 2

2 large beets (about 11 oz),
  chopped into chunks
  or wedges
1 red onion, quartered
2 tbsp olive oil
2 tbsp balsamic vinegar
2 ripe figs, quartered
2 tbsp coarsely chopped
  walnuts or hazelnuts
2 oz feta
Generous handful of basil
  leaves, torn

Preheat the oven to 400°F. Spread the beets and onion on a baking pan, drizzle over the oil and vinegar and season with salt and pepper. Cover the pan with foil and place it in the oven. After 20 minutes stir in the figs and walnuts and return the pan to the oven, uncovered, for another 20 minutes. When the mixture has cooled, crumble the feta over it and stir in the basil.

Tip: wear rubber gloves when you peel and cut the beets as it will stain your fingers.

- **CALORIES** 210
- PROTEIN 4G
- FAT 14G
- FIBER 3G
- CARBS 18G

Crunchy red coleslaw with minute steak

Serves 2

2 small steaks, such as skirt
  or sirloin, beaten thinner
½ small red cabbage, outer
  leaves removed
1 carrot
1 red apple
4 spring onions, finely
  sliced
1 tbsp olive oil
1 tbsp cider vinegar
2 tbsp mayonnaise

Season the steaks with salt and pepper (or a sprinkle of steak seasoning). Finely shred the cabbage and place it in a bowl. Grate the carrot and apple into the bowl and add the spring onions. Make a dressing by whisking together the oil, vinegar, and mayonnaise and stir it through the cabbage mixture. Heat a griddle pan and cook the steaks to your liking. Slice them diagonally and serve them with the coleslaw.

- **CALORIES** 430
- PROTEIN 23G
- FAT 31G
- FIBER 5G
- CARBS 14G

Main Meals

These are more substantial recipes suited to occasions when you have extra time for cooking, perhaps on the weekend or when family and friends are around.

As you know, we Blood Sugar dieters are trying to avoid using starchy carbohydrates wherever possible. Fortunately, there are lots of tasty and filling alternatives so you should be able to keep everyone happy. Cauliflower mash is a brilliant substitute for mashed potato, astonishingly low in starchy carbohydrate. Beans and lentils are great for thickening casseroles and stews. And there are all sorts of healthy toppings you can use on bakes, pies, and gratins—those ideal one-pot meals, ready the moment you pull them out of the oven.

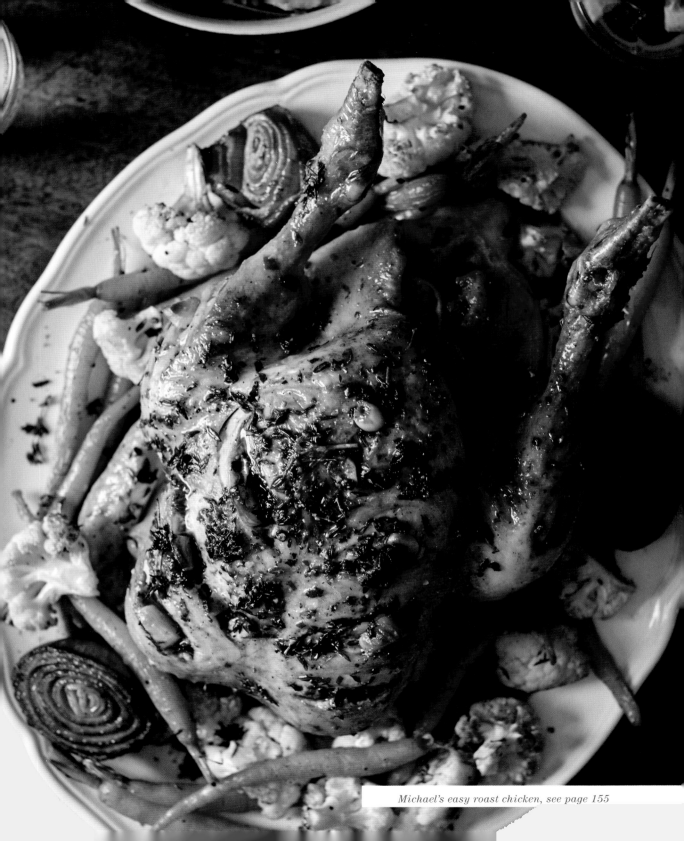

Michael's easy roast chicken, see page 155

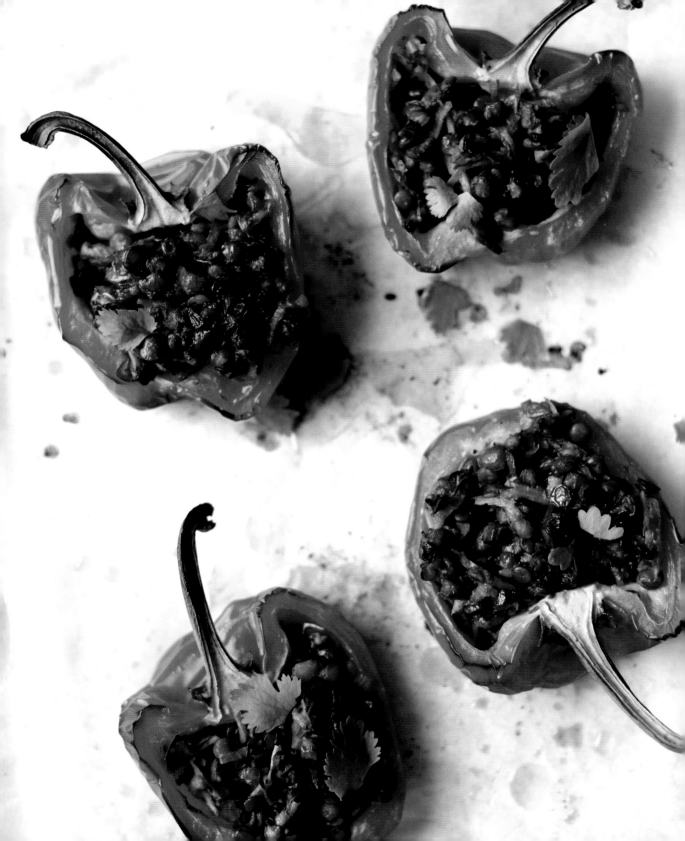

Spicy stuffed red pepper

This recipe was contributed by our great friends Drs. Rajsingh and Rai who specialize in healthy Indian food. The dahl stuffing has an exotic nutty flavor, spicy but not hot, and works well eaten hot or cold.

Serves 2

2 tbsp vegetable or olive oil
2 medium onions, chopped
9-10 oz package
  microwaveable Puy
  lentils, or 1 (14-oz) can
  green lentils, rinsed and
  drained
3-4 garlic cloves, diced, or
  2 tsp garlic paste
1¾ inch fresh ginger, diced,
  or 1 tsp ginger paste
2 bay leaves
2 cinnamon sticks
2 cardamom pods
1 tsp ground cumin
  or seeds
1 chile, diced, or 1 tsp
  red pepper flakes (to taste)
Handful of cilantro,
  chopped
Juice of 1 lime
2 large red bell peppers,
  halved lengthwise and
  seeded

Preheat the oven to 350°F. Heat 1 tbsp of the oil in a saucepan and gently cook the onions for about 5 minutes, or until they start to turn golden brown. Meanwhile, put the lentils, garlic, ginger, bay leaves, cinnamon sticks, cardamoms, cumin, and chile in a medium bowl and mix them. Season with salt and pepper.

When the onions are ready, add the lentil mixture and simmer on low heat for 8 to 10 minutes, before stirring in the cilantro and lime juice. Then fill the bell pepper halves with the mixture and place them on a greased baking sheet with the open side facing up. Drizzle the remaining 1 tbsp oil over them, cover them with foil, and bake for 10 minutes. Remove the foil and bake them for another 10 minutes.

Tips: with the flat of a knife gently crush the cardamom pod to release the flavor. If you prefer you can prepare the green lentils from scratch, using ½ cup dried lentils (see page 197).

- **CALORIES** 240
- PROTEIN 6G
- FAT 13G
- FIBER 8G
- CARBS 28G

Easy Bolognese

This is a great foolproof Bolognese, and makes a fairly large batch from which you can save or freeze portions to create all sorts of other dishes—see no-pasta beef "lasagna" and chili con carne (opposite).

Serves 6

1 onion, finely diced
1 tbsp olive oil
1 lb ground beef (or commercial vegetarian mixture)
1 garlic clove, diced
2 heaping tsp dried oregano
2 medium carrots, grated
2 (14-oz) cans chopped tomatoes
1 beef stock cube
2 tbsp tomato puree
½ tbsp Worcestershire sauce
½ tsp red pepper flakes (to taste)
3 bay leaves

In a medium casserole, gently cook the onion in the olive oil until it is golden brown—about 5 minutes. Add the beef, garlic, and oregano and cook until the meat is lightly browned.

Stir in the carrots, tomatoes, stock cube, tomato puree, Worcestershire sauce, red pepper flakes, and bay leaves, cover the pan, and simmer for about an hour, stirring occasionally and adding a little water if it's looking dry. Serve with steamed or boiled finely sliced cabbage, zucchini noodles (see page 107), or konjac noodles (see page 198).

- **CALORIES** 170
- PROTEIN 17G
- FAT 9G
- FIBER 1G
- CARBS 5G

Chili con carne

Use the Bolognese (left) as a base and simply add these extra ingredients, adjusting the proportions according to how much Bolognese you are converting. So if you have half left, use half the quantities below.

Serves 6

1 tbsp cocoa powder
  (not drinking chocolate
  which is full of sugar!)
1 tsp ground cumin
1 tsp ground coriander
1 red bell pepper, seeded
  and finely diced
7 oz mushrooms, sliced
1 (14-oz) can kidney beans
  or black beans, rinsed and
  drained
1 tsp diced chile, or red
  pepper flakes (to taste)
Sour cream, to serve

Stir the cocoa powder, cumin, coriander, bell pepper, mushrooms, beans, and chile into the Bolognese base, cover the pan and simmer for 15 to 20 minutes, adding water if it starts to dry out. Serve with a dollop of sour cream on top, and steamed finely sliced cabbage or cauliflower rice (see page 98).

- **CALORIES** 260
- PROTEIN 23G
- FAT 1G
- FIBER 7G
- CARBS 19G

No-pasta beef "lasagna"

A delicious low-carb lasagna, in which the sheets of pasta are replaced with red cabbage leaves. Our daughter was horrified at the thought of cabbage in a lasagna, but it works surprisingly well. Try it and see.

Serves 6

4 x portions of Bolognese
  sauce (see recipe opposite)
4 oz outer leaves of red
  cabbage (or white)

For the white sauce:
9 oz ricotta
1 cup plus 2 tbsp crème
  fraîche
¼ cup grated Parmesan
4 oz spinach
½ tsp nutmeg
4 oz grated Cheddar

Preheat the oven to 300°F. In a pan, heat the Bolognese sauce and transfer it to a large baking dish. Cut each cabbage leaf in half and remove the tough central stalk, taking care not to tear the rest of the leaf. Place a single layer of cabbage leaves over the Bolognese sauce, overlapping them slightly to keep the Bolognese separate from the creamy sauce to be added next.

Mix the ricotta, crème fraîche, and Parmesan in a bowl and stir in the spinach. Add the nutmeg and some ground black pepper, then dollop the mixture over the layer of red cabbage. Sprinkle the Cheddar on top and bake for 30 to 40 minutes.

- **CALORIES** 500
- PROTEIN 29G
- FAT 38G
- FIBER 2G
- CARBS 10G

Michael's Thai fish cakes

Michael has whipped these fish cakes together with great speed and in large quantities for several parties, but they are also perfect for a light meal. They have a great texture and an exotic flavor and, because we use chia seeds rather than flour or bread crumbs to bind the mixture, they are less starchy and more nutritious.

Serves 2

For the sweet and sour dipping sauce:
2-3 tsp sweet chili sauce (see page 175)
1 tsp Thai fish sauce
1 tsp cider vinegar
2 tsp water
1 tbsp very finely diced cucumber

7 oz white fish fillets, skinned and cut into chunks
1 egg
2 tsp Thai red curry paste (to taste)
½ tbsp Thai fish sauce
¼ tsp lime zest, finely shredded
1 spring onion, finely diced (set aside 1 tsp for the dipping sauce)
1 tbsp finely chopped cilantro
2 tsp chia seeds
1 tbsp coconut or rapeseed oil

Put the chili sauce, fish sauce, vinegar, water, and cucumber in a small saucepan and bring them to a boil, then simmer for about 1 minute. Pour the sauce into 2 small bowls.

Drain any fluid from the fish and blend it with the egg, curry paste, fish sauce, lime zest, spring onion, cilantro, chia seeds, and oil either in a food processor or blender until you have a slightly coarse texture. Place the mixture in the fridge for 10 minutes to firm it up a little, then divide it into 4 pieces. Flatten each piece into a patty.

Heat the oil in a frying pan and fry the patties on medium heat for 2 to 3 minutes on each side, or until they are golden brown. Serve with the dipping sauce and cabbage stir-fried Chinese style (see page 169) or Swiss chard stir-fried with garlic (see pg 168).

- **CALORIES** 130
- PROTEIN 21G
- FAT 3G
- FIBER 0G
- CARBS 4G

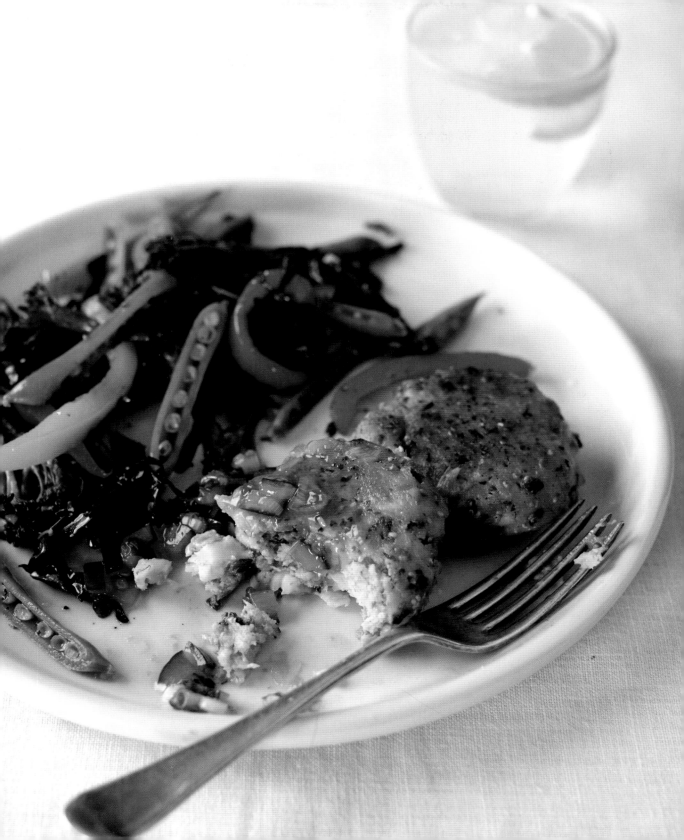

Pork steaks in mustard sauce

These are wonderfully quick and easy to prepare. The creamy mustard sauce soaks up the juices and complements the pork deliciously.

Serves 2

*2 boneless pork steaks
  or boneless chops
½ tbsp olive oil
2 generous tsp mustard
  (grainy or Dijon)
2 level tbsp crème fraîche
Small handful of parsley,
  chopped*

Fry the pork steaks in the oil in a small frying pan for 15 to 20 minutes, or until the juices do not run pink. Take the pan off the heat, allow the meat to cool for a few minutes, and then add the mustard and crème fraîche, stirring them into the juices. Season and scatter with the parsley.

Serve with 2 tbsp cooked grains such as quinoa or bulgur wheat to soak up the juices (see page 99) and green vegetables.

- **CALORIES** 290
- PROTEIN 25G
- FAT 20G
- FIBER 0G
- CARBS 2G

Bulgur wheat risotto with chicken and artichokes

Bulgur wheat is a whole grain cereal which has been parboiled, allowing it to be cooked more quickly, and retain a fairly high fiber content. This "risotto" is also an excellent way to use up leftover chicken.

Serves 2

1 onion, finely chopped
1 large garlic clove, diced
   or squeezed
1 tbsp olive oil
¼ cup bulgur wheat
½-1 red chile, diced, or
   ½ tsp red pepper flakes
   (to taste)
1 bay leaf
1 red bell pepper, seeded
   and sliced
1 cup plus 2 tbsp chicken
   or vegetable stock
5 oz cooked leftover
   chicken, chopped (about
1 medium chicken breast)
2 heaping tbsp artichokes
   (from a jar or can),
   quartered
Large handful of cilantro
   or parsley, coarsely
   chopped

Gently cook the onions and garlic in the oil in a saucepan. Add the bulgur wheat, chile, bay leaf, and bell pepper and cover with about ¾ inch of stock. Put on the lid and let simmer for 20 to 25 minutes, or until most of the fluid has been absorbed and the bulgur wheat is al dente. Check every now and again and add extra stock if it is looking dry.

Then stir the chicken into the pan, along with the artichokes, for the last 5 to 10 minutes of cooking. Season and stir in half the cilantro, reserving the rest to garnish.

Tip: this also works really well if you swap the chicken for 2 oz fried sliced halloumi.

- **CALORIES** 330
- PROTEIN 22G
- FAT 12G
- FIBER 2G
- CARBS 35G

Garlic and rosemary fried lamb

Full of Mediterranean flavors and so easy to prepare, this lamb is delicious served with quinoa. Quinoa is great for occasional use on the Blood Sugar Diet as it has far more protein and fiber than rice and therefore a lower impact on blood sugar (see page 99).

Serves 2

1 garlic clove
2 sprigs rosemary,
  leaves only
1 tbsp olive oil
Squeeze of lemon juice
2 lamb chops, or medium
  lamb steaks
⅓ cup quinoa (the darker
  variety if available)
¾ cup chicken or
  vegetable stock
¼ cucumber, cut in half
  lengthwise and seeded

Use a mortar and pestle (or a spoon in a bowl) to crush together the garlic and rosemary leaves with a drizzle of oil and the lemon juice. Place the lamb chops in a dish, pour on the marinade and spread it over the surface of the meat.

Put the quinoa in a small saucepan, cover it with ¼ to ¾ inch of stock and bring it to a boil. Then immediately put the lid on and turn down the heat. Simmer for 10 minutes, or until the liquid has been absorbed. Turn off the heat and let it steam with the lid on for another 10 minutes. Dice the cucumber finely and put it aside to add to the quinoa before serving.

When the quinoa is nearly ready, season the lamb, then fry it on both sides in a drizzle of oil in a nonstick pan until it is slightly browned. Serve the lamb with greens or green beans and a couple of tablespoons of quinoa, and pour over any juices remaining in the pan.

- **CALORIES 330**
- PROTEIN 29G
- FAT 16G
- FIBER 2G
- CARBS 18G

Chicken korma

An old favorite that went out of fashion in the days of low-fat diets but, hurrah, is now back on the menu.

Serves 2

2 tbsp oil

2 onions, one finely chopped, the other sliced into rings

2 garlic cloves, finely chopped

¼ inch fresh ginger, finely chopped

1 tsp garam masala

½ tsp cayenne pepper

Seeds from 4 cardamom pods

1 tsp turmeric

4 small boneless, skinless chicken thighs, or 2 small chicken breasts, chopped into ¼-¾ inch chunks

¾ cup coconut milk or full-fat plain Greek yogurt

2 tbsp ground almonds

½ medium cauliflower, grated

Handful of cilantro, coarsely chopped

Heat 1 tbsp of the oil in an ovenproof casserole or pan and fry the finely chopped onions, garlic, and ginger over medium heat for 2 to 3 minutes. Add the ginger, garam masala, cayenne, cardamom, and turmeric and cook for 1 minute more.

Add the chicken and cook for 2 to 3 minutes, then pour in the coconut milk and almonds and simmer on the stove top for 20 minutes. Alternatively, put the casserole in an oven preheated to 300°F for 20 minutes.

Meanwhile, heat the remaining 1 tbsp oil in a nonstick frying pan and fry the onion rings for 5 to 10 minutes, or until they are browned, turning them frequently. Remove the onion rings with a slotted spoon and place them on paper towels.

When the curry is nearly ready, fry the grated cauliflower gently in the oil remaining from the fried onions for 5 minutes.

Season the curry and stir in the cilantro. Place the cauliflower rice on the plate, add the curry, scatter the fried onions on top, and serve with 4 oz of green beans.

- **CALORIES** 340
- PROTEIN 28G
- FAT 19G
- FIBER 5G
- CARBS 17G

Thai red curry

A gently spicy, aromatic Thai curry, with a creamy sweetness thanks to the coconut milk, and quick to make if you use a store-bought curry paste.

Serves 2

1 tbsp olive oil
1 large boneless, skinless chicken breast, sliced
½ onion, chopped
1 large garlic clove, diced
¾ inch fresh ginger, diced
3-4 heaping tsp Thai red curry paste
1 red bell pepper, seeded and sliced
1½ cups canned coconut milk
½ tbsp Thai fish sauce
½ tsp lime zest or kaffir lime leaves (optional)
½ cauliflower, grated
Generous handful of haricots verts

Heat the oil in a wok or wide-based saucepan and fry the chicken and onion. When they begin to brown, add the garlic, ginger, and curry paste. Fry gently for a few minutes, then add the bell pepper, coconut milk, fish sauce, and lime zest and cook for 15 minutes.

Meanwhile, prepare the cauliflower rice (see page 98). A few minutes before the end of cooking time, throw the green vegetables in the pan.

Tips: you can use shrimp or tofu instead of chicken. Kaffir lime leaves can be bought fresh and kept in the freezer.

- **CALORIES** 300
- PROTEIN 4G
- FAT 25G
- FIBER 2G
- CARBS 14G

Smoked mackerel and mushroom frittata

Serves 2

3 eggs
½ cup cottage cheese
2 tbsp grated Parmesan
½ tbsp olive oil
2 oz mushrooms, sliced
2 spring onions, chopped
2 peppered mackerel fillets, flaked
2 large handfuls baby spinach, chopped
½-1 tsp red pepper flakes, (optional)

Preheat the broiler to high. Whisk the eggs in a bowl with the cottage cheese and Parmesan. Season with a pinch of salt and plenty of black pepper and set aside.

Heat the oil in an ovenproof frying pan or omelet pan. Fry the mushrooms for 3 to 4 minutes, then add the spring onions and mackerel and cook for another 2 minutes. Stir in the spinach and cook it until it has just wilted. Make sure the mixture is spread evenly over the pan, then pour over the eggs and a sprinkling of red pepper flakes, if using, and cook gently for 4 to 5 minutes on the stove top.

Put the pan under the broiler for about 4 minutes, until the eggs have set. Serve warm with a green leafy salad.

- **CALORIES** 380
- PROTEIN 27G
- FAT 29G
- FIBER 1G
- CARBS 2G

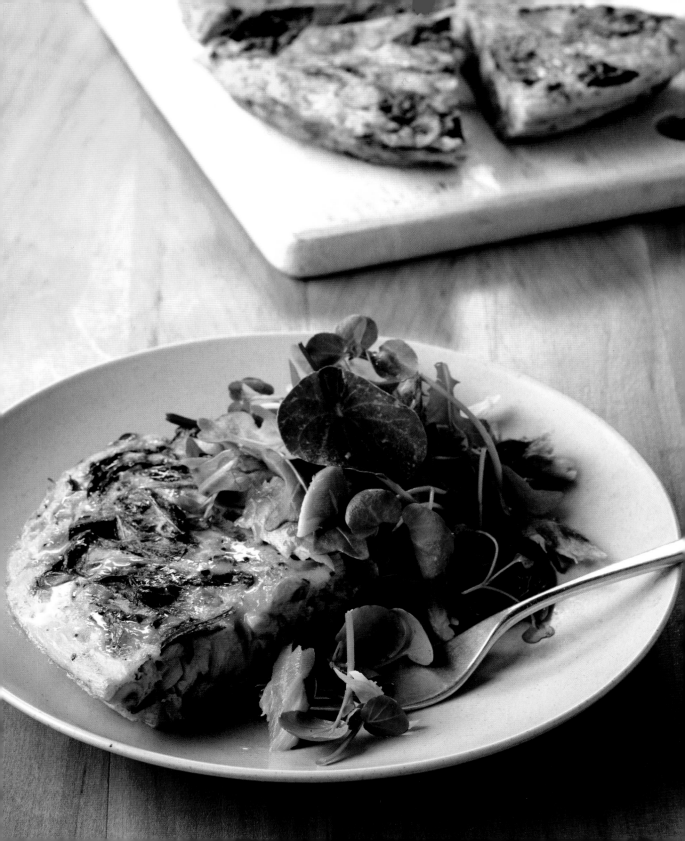

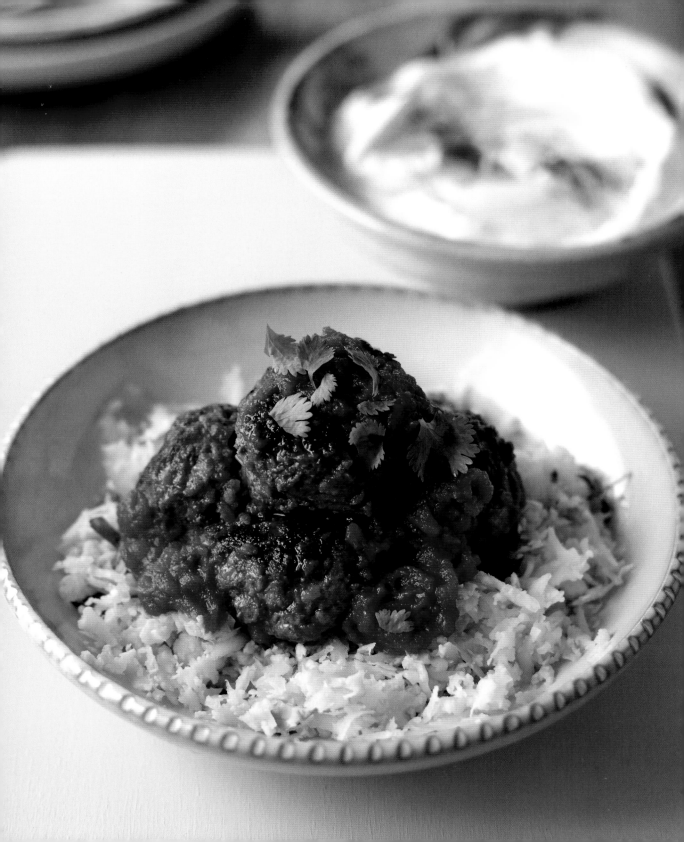

Moroccan meatballs in tomato sauce

Serves 6

14 oz ground lamb or beef
1 onion, diced (half very
   finely for the meatballs)
2 small garlic cloves,
   finely diced
1 egg
2 tbsp olive oil
1¾ cups canned chopped
   tomatoes
½ tsp paprika
½ tsp ground cumin
½ tsp red pepper flakes
   or chili paste
Handful of cilantro or
   parsley, chopped

Vigorously mix the ground meat with the finely diced onion, garlic, and egg in a bowl. Season with salt and black pepper. Roll the mixture into about 16 plum-size balls and place them in the fridge to firm up while you are preparing the sauce.

Fry the rest of the onion gently in 1 tbsp of the oil until it is golden brown, then add the tomatoes, paprika, cumin, and red pepper flakes. Simmer gently for 15 to 20 minutes.

Heat the remaining 1 tbsp oil in a large frying pan and fry the meatballs. When they are browned, add them to the sauce to cook through. Season to taste; stir in half the cilantro and garnish with the rest. Serve with cauliflower rice (adds 30 calories; see page 98)

Tip: alternatively, you can make these into burgers, adding the spices to the ground meat instead, and serve them with a salad.

- **CALORIES** 390
- PROTEIN 29G
- FAT 28G
- FIBER 2G
- CARBS 8G

Chinese duck with green "pancakes"

Okay, I concede that it is pushing it to call lettuce a pancake . . . but for years we felt guilty eating duck pancakes because of the high-fat content in duck, only to realize we have been worrying about the wrong thing. It's the starchy pancakes we should avoid. The sugar in the hoisin sauce is absorbed slowly as part of the meal, so is not of much significance here.

Serves 2

2 duck legs
1 tbsp soy sauce
½ tbsp sesame oil
  (optional)
1 small cucumber, cut in
  half lengthwise and
  seeded
6 spring onions
Hoisin sauce (1 tsp per
  "pancake")
Romaine or Boston lettuce

Place the duck in an oven pan, score the surface with a sharp knife, and rub soy sauce into the skin. Drizzle with the oil, if using. Leave the duck to marinate while the oven heats to 400°F. As soon as you place the duck in the oven, reduce the temperature to 300°F and roast it for an hour, turning and basting it regularly. Chop the cucumber and spring onions into matchsticks and place them on 2 separate plates.

The duck is ready when the flesh easily comes away from the bone. Use a spoon and fork to shred it and serve on a plate with the vegetables, lettuce "pancakes," and a bowl of hoisin sauce.

- CALORIES 340
- PROTEIN 13G
- FAT 35G
- FIBER 1G
- CARBS 5G

Low-carb pizza

Serves 1

3 oz celeriac (celery root),
  peeled and grated
2 tbsp cream cheese
1 tbsp grated Cheddar
1 egg, beaten
1 tsp olive oil
3 tbsp tomato pizza paste,
  or tomato puree
2 mozzarella balls, torn
Handful of basil leaves,
  shredded
Handful of black olives
  chopped

Preheat the oven to 400°F. Place the celeriac in a bowl, add the cheeses and mix in the egg with some black pepper. Line a baking pan with parchment paper brushed with a little oil. Shape the celeriac mixture into a circle on the paper and bake for 15 minutes.

Remove the base from the oven and allow it to cool for a minute or so before spreading on the tomato paste. Then dot it with the mozzarella, basil, and olives and return it to the oven for another 4 to 5 minutes.

Tips: use grated cauliflower instead of celeriac for the base. Add anchovies, spinach, feta, or the topping of your choice. You can bake several of the bases at a time and store them in the freezer.

- CALORIES 490
- PROTEIN 30G
- FAT 38G
- FIBER 4G
- CARBS 6G

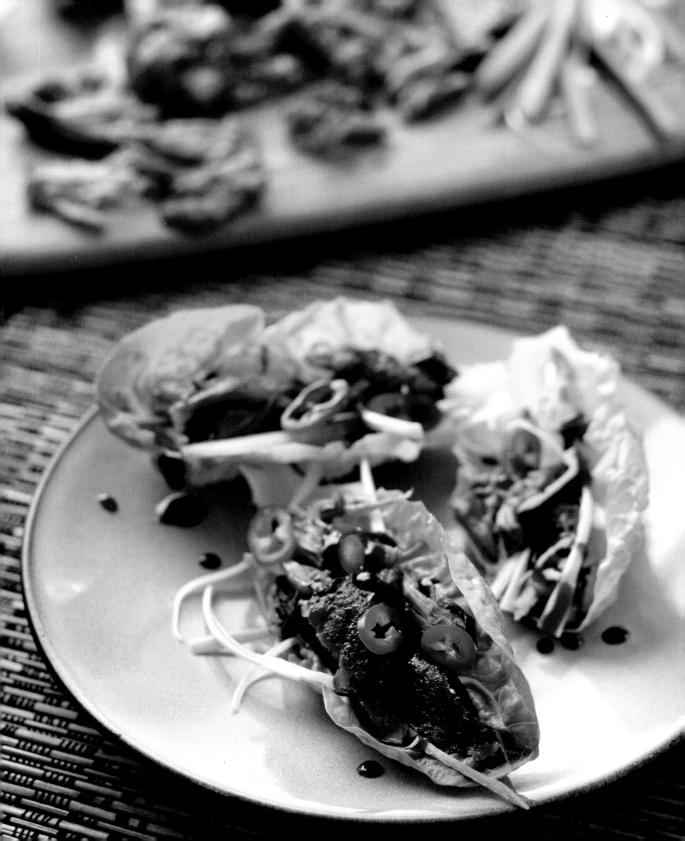

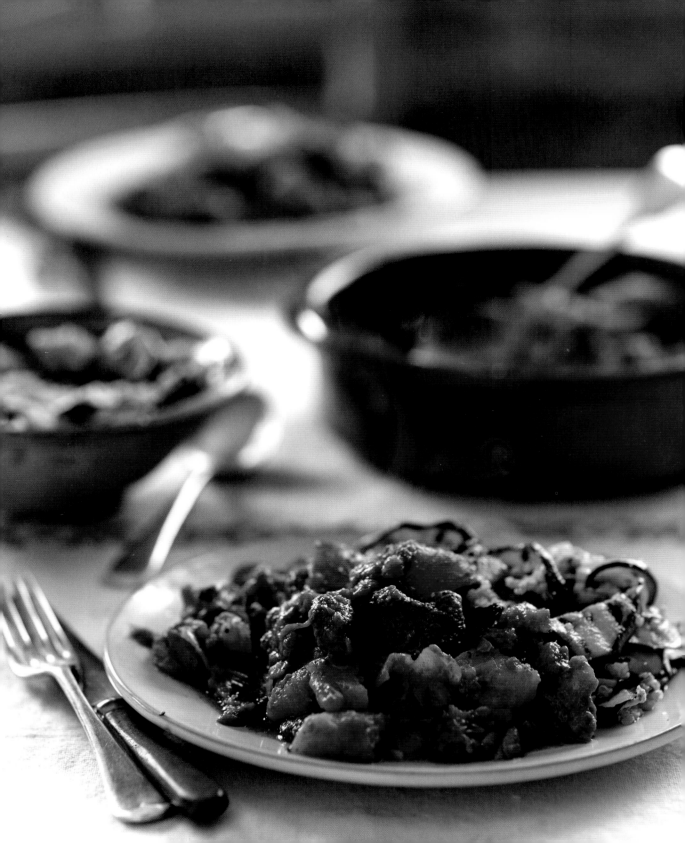

Lamb tagine

This is one of the easiest stews to make, despite the long list of ingredients. It really is a case of chuck it in and let it cook. It is full of North African flavors, the sweetness of the apricots melding deliciously with the spices and the tang of lemon.

Serves 4

14 oz stewing lamb, diced
2 tbsp olive oil
1 onion, diced
1 red bell pepper, seeded
  and diced
3 garlic cloves, diced
1½ inches fresh ginger,
  diced
2 tsp turmeric
3 tsp paprika
2 tsp ground cumin
1 tsp ground cilantro
½-1 tsp red pepper flakes,
  fresh chile, or chili paste
2 oz dried apricots,
  chopped
2 cups plus 2 tbsp chicken
  or vegetable stock
Juice of half a lemon
7 oz butternut squash
  pieces (you can buy them
  ready prepared)

Preheat the oven to 300°F. Put all the ingredients, except the lemon juice and butternut squash, in a casserole. Cover and cook it in the oven for 2 hours, checking it occasionally and topping up the stock if necessary. Add the lemon juice and butternut squash and cook for another 1 to 2 hours. Again, add extra water if it looks dry.

Before serving, add another squeeze of lemon and some salt and black pepper. Serve with quinoa (see page 99) and a green vegetable such as steamed zucchini noodles.

- **CALORIES** 420
- PROTEIN 32G
- FAT 27G
- FIBER 3G
- CARBS 16G

Hungarian goulash

A rich, thick beef soup from Hungary, ideal for warming up a dark wintery evening. It looks like a lot of ingredients, but it is very easy to assemble.

Serves 4

2 tbsp olive oil
2 medium onions, chopped
1 garlic clove, diced
4 oz baby carrots or carrots cut into batons (short sticks)
14 oz stewing beef, diced
1 green bell pepper, seeded and chopped
1 red bell pepper, seeded and chopped
2 tbsp paprika
1 tsp nutmeg
3 tsp mixed herbs
2 bay leaves
1 tbsp cornstarch
3 tbsp tomato puree
¾ cup beef stock
2 (14-oz) cans chopped tomatoes
¾ cup red wine
1 tbsp Worcestershire sauce
1 tbsp cider vinegar
⅔ cup sour cream
Generous handful of parsley, chopped

Preheat the oven to 300°F. Heat the oil in an ovenproof casserole and gently fry the onion, garlic, and carrots till softened (7 to 8 minutes). Add the meat and stir to brown it all over.

Add the bell peppers, paprika, nutmeg, mixed herbs, and bay leaves, season with salt and pepper, and cook for 2 minutes. Scatter over the cornstarch and mix it in well before adding the tomato puree, stock, tomatoes, wine, Worcestershire sauce, and vinegar. Bring it to a simmer, then transfer the casserole to the oven and cook for 3 to 4 hours, checking that it has not dried out and stirring occasionally.

Serve the goulash in a bowl with a dollop of sour cream and fresh parsley. You could also serve it with roasted cauliflower (see page 165).

- **CALORIES** 350
- PROTEIN 28G
- FAT 15G
- FIBER 3G
- CARBS 27G

Spanish chicken with chorizo and beans

Serves 2

3 tbsp olive oil
2 large or 4 small boneless,
  skinless chicken thighs
1 onion, chopped
2 chorizo sausages,
  chopped
1 tsp thyme
Sprig of rosemary
2 garlic cloves, chopped
3-3½ oz olives, drained
⅔ cup chicken stock
1 (14-oz) can chopped
  tomatoes
Juice of half a lemon
1 (14-oz) can navy or
  cannellini beans, rinsed
  and drained

Preheat the oven to 325°F. In a heavy casserole, heat 1 tbsp of the oil and brown the chicken all over. Meanwhile, in a separate pan, heat 1 tbsp of the oil and gently fry the onion, chorizo, thyme, rosemary, and garlic for about 5 minutes, then transfer the mixture to the main casserole. Add the olives, stock, tomatoes, and lemon juice and bring to a boil. Then put the lid on and place the casserole in the oven for 50 to 60 minutes. Serve with vegetables such as steamed cavolo nero or steamed or panfried zucchini.

Tip: to add extra flavor use olives stuffed with anchovies (assuming you don't get carried away like me and eat them first).

- **CALORIES** 540
- PROTEIN 38G
- FAT 24G
- FIBER 16G
- CARBS 47G

Piri piri chicken

This is quite a spicy dish—piri piri means "pepper pepper" in Swahili—but you can adjust how much flavoring you add, particularly if you make your own.

Serves 2

2 tbsp olive oil
1 tbsp cider vinegar
3 garlic cloves
1-2 tsp piri piri flavoring
  (or make your own: see
  tip)
2 medium boneless,
  skinless chicken thighs
2 red bell peppers,
  seeded and sliced
4 oz small tomatoes
1 fennel bulb, cut into
  quarters through the base
1 lime (or lemon), cut
  into quarters

To make the marinade, mix the oil, vinegar, garlic, and piri piri. Place the chicken in a large baking dish and pour on the marinade. Leave it at room temperature for 1 hour, or in the fridge for 4 hours.

Preheat the oven to 350°F. Add the bell peppers, tomatoes, fennel, and lime to the chicken and stir them into the marinade with some salt and a generous amount of black pepper. Bake the chicken for 40 to 50 minutes. Serve it with a small portion of brown rice, lentils, or quinoa (2 tbsp maximum per person) and a green salad.

Tip: to make your own piri piri, mix 1 tsp paprika, 1 tsp dried oregano, and 1 to 2 fresh chiles, seeded and diced (or 1 to 2 tsp red pepper flakes).

- **CALORIES** 270
- PROTEIN 12G
- FAT 18G
- FIBER 4G
- CARBS 13G

Coq au vin

A classic French dish made with braised chicken and a rich red wine and mushroom sauce. Served here with cauliflower mash to mop up the flavors in the gravy.

Serves 4

1 tbsp olive oil
4 chicken legs
10 shallots
2 oz pancetta or smoked
  bacon
1 garlic clove, crushed
7 oz white or cremini
  mushrooms, sliced
2 tsp dried thyme
2-3 bay leaves
1 tbsp cornstarch
1½ cups red wine
1¼ cups chicken stock
Bouquet garni
1 carrot, cut into batons
  (short sticks)
Handful of parsley, chopped

Preheat the oven to 350°F. Heat the oil in a large ovenproof pan and fry the chicken, turning it frequently, until it is golden all over. Add the shallots, pancetta, garlic, mushrooms, thyme, and bay leaves and let them cook gently for 5 minutes, then scatter over the cornstarch. Add the wine and stock, bouquet garni, and carrot and stir well. Transfer the dish to the oven and cook for 30 minutes.

If the sauce is too runny, pour some of it into a pan, bring it to a boil, and let it simmer uncovered to reduce it. Scatter with the parsley and serve it with cauliflower mash (see page 196).

- **CALORIES** 510
- PROTEIN 40G
- FAT 28G
- FIBER 2G
- CARBS 10G

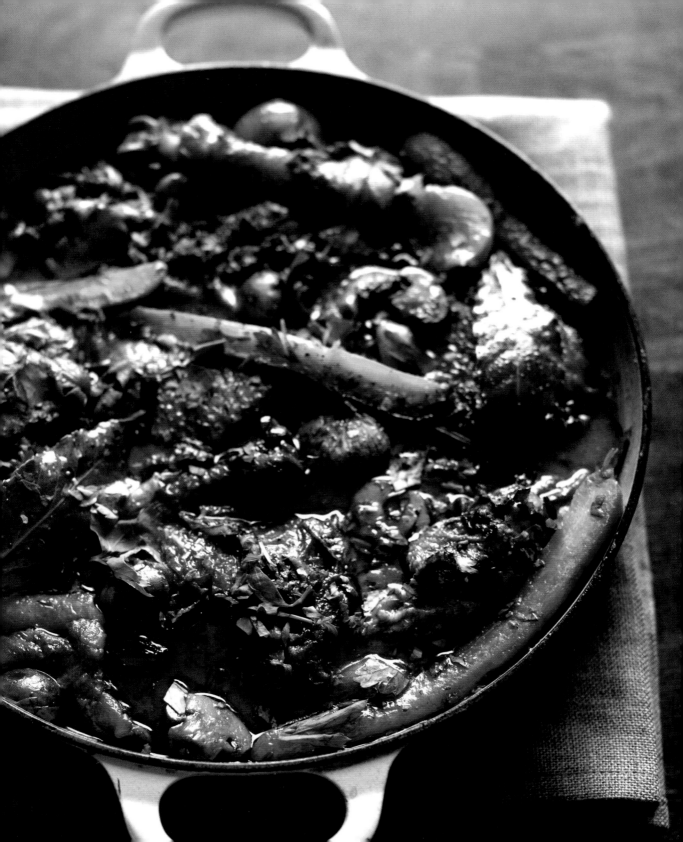

Skinny cottage pie

Perfect comfort food. Swapping the starchy mashed potato topping for cauliflower mash makes all the difference.

Serves 6

1 tbsp olive oil
1 small onion, diced
1 lb ground beef
2 garlic cloves, sliced
1-2 tsp dried thyme
1 (14 oz) can chopped
  tomatoes
1 beef or vegetable stock
  cube or 1 tsp
  Worcestershire sauce
2 carrots, diced
2 bay leaves

For the cauliflower mash:
1 medium cauliflower
3 oz Cheddar, grated
2 tsp olive oil
2 tbsp full-fat fromage frais
  or sour cream
2 spring onions, finely
  chopped
1 tsp grated Parmesan

Preheat the oven to 400°F. Heat the oil in a saucepan and gently cook the onion until it is golden, then add the beef, garlic, and thyme. When the meat is cooked through, stir in the tomatoes, stock cube, carrots, bay leaves, and enough water to cover the mixture. Put the lid on and simmer for about an hour.

Meanwhile, to make the mash, chop the cauliflower into pieces about ¾ inch in diameter, then steam or boil them for 8 to 10 minutes, or until they are soft. Mash the cauliflower vigorously. Note that it won't form the creamy solid texture of mashed potatoes). Add the cheese, oil, fromage frais, and spring onions and mix well.

Put the meat in an ovenproof dish, dollop the mash on top, then scatter over the Parmesan. Bake the pie on the middle rack of the oven for 20 to 30 minutes, or until it is crispy on top.

Tips: to meld the flavors, cook the ground beef mixture gently for an hour if you have time, stirring and topping up with water or stock as needed. To improve the texture of the mash, you can add half a 14 oz can of chickpeas (rinsed and drained first). This will add 150 calories to the dish.

- **CALORIES** 310
- PROTEIN 23G
- FAT 21G
- FIBER 3G
- CARBS 8G

Creamy fish bake

Serves 6

1 tbsp olive oil
4 shallots, or 2 small
  onions, chopped
3 garlic cloves, crushed
2 tbsp butter
¾ cup heavy cream
1 tbsp crème fraîche
1 tbsp finely chopped
  chives or spring
  onion
1 tbsp finely chopped
  parsley
1 tbsp finely chopped
  tarragon, or 1 tsp dried
¼ cup white wine
1 tbsp lemon juice
2-3 eggs
1 small celeriac (celery
  root), peeled and chopped
14 oz mixed fish (such as
  haddock, cod, and smoked
  salmon), cut into chunks
2 oz Cheddar, grated

Preheat the oven to 400°F. Heat the oil in a frying pan and gently cook the shallots and garlic for 4 to 5 minutes, or until they have softened. In a separate pan, melt half the butter, then pour in the heavy cream and crème fraîche, and heat the mixture without letting it boil. Add the shallots and garlic together with the chives, parsley, and tarragon, followed by the wine. Season the sauce with a pinch of salt and black pepper, and lemon juice to taste.

Meanwhile, boil the eggs in a pan of water for 6 to 7 minutes, then plunge them into cold water to cool them. Peel and coarsely chop them before stirring them into the sauce. Place the celeriac in a pan of boiling water and cook it for 6 to 8 minutes, or until it is tender, then mash it with the remaining butter.

Stir the fish pieces into the sauce and bring it to a boil, then transfer the mixture to an ovenproof dish, and spread the mash over the top. Sprinkle with the grated cheese and bake for about 15 minutes.

- **CALORIES** 360
- PROTEIN 19G
- FAT 29G
- FIBER 3G
- CARBS 3G

Skinny eggplant "lasagna"

Inspired by a great recipe from Cherianne on the Blood Sugar Diet website in which we use thinly sliced eggplant instead of zucchini as it keeps its texture better. An excellent low-cal, low-carb Mediterranean-style vegetarian meal for anyone missing pasta.

Serves 4

2 oz fresh spinach, or frozen and thawed

2 oz Parmesan, grated

4 oz cottage cheese (or ricotta, but note it has more calories and less protein)

½ red bell pepper, seeded and finely chopped

7 oz mushrooms, chopped

1 large garlic clove, crushed

2 tsp dried oregano

1 tsp dried basil

1 cup plus 2 tbsp tomato sauce

1 tbsp olive oil

7 oz eggplant, sliced lengthwise in very thin strips

12 cherry tomatoes, halved, or 6 larger tomatoes, chopped

2 oz Cheddar, grated

Preheat the oven to 400°F. Finely chop the spinach and mix it with the Parmesan and cottage cheese in a bowl, and season to taste. Place the bell pepper and mushrooms in a separate bowl along with the garlic, oregano, basil, tomato sauce, and oil. Season well.

Spread half the tomato and vegetable mixture over the bottom of a rectangular ovenproof dish or pan, followed by alternating layers of sliced eggplant and the cheese and spinach mix. The last layer should be eggplant. Pour the rest of the tomato mix over the top and dot with the tomatoes. Cover the dish with foil and bake for approximately 30 minutes, or until the eggplant feels soft and thoroughly cooked.

Remove the foil and sprinkle grated cheese over the top of the lasagna. Put it back in the oven for another 10 to 15 minutes, or until the cheese has melted and browned. Serve with a crunchy green salad.

Tip: you could add Quorn or ground meat to the tomato mix if desired.

- **CALORIES** 200
- PROTEIN 14G
- FAT 13G
- FIBER 3G
- CARBS 7G

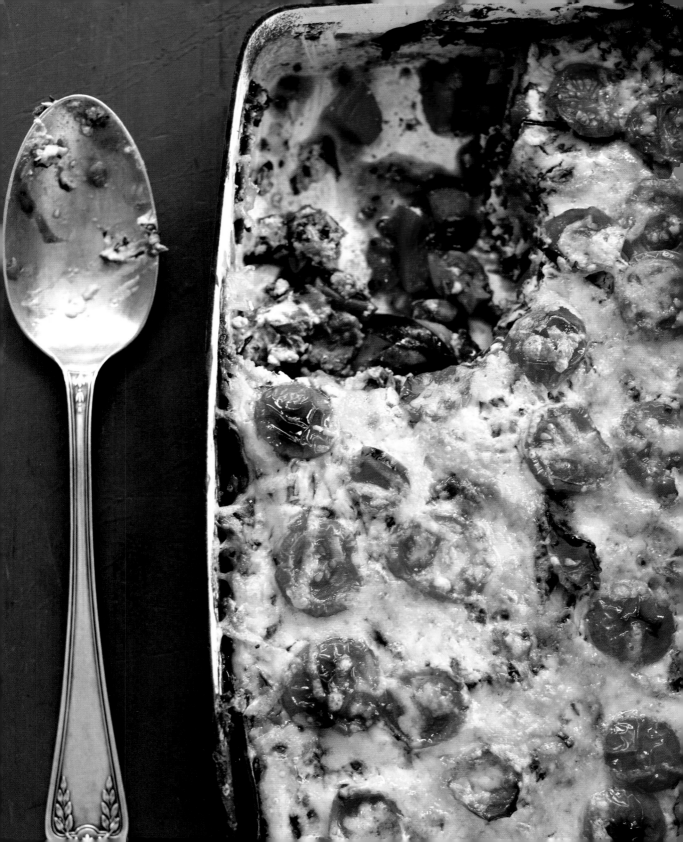

Chicken and mushroom "pie"

A yummy meal in one dish, just without the pastry.

Serves 6

2 small onions, diced
2 tbsp olive oil
8 boneless, skinless chicken
 thighs, or 6 medium
 chicken breasts, cut into
 chunks
7 oz mushrooms, sliced
½ tsp ground nutmeg
1 tbsp cornstarch
½ cup chicken stock (made
 with ¼ stock cube)
2 heaping tbsp crème
 fraîche
2 tsp mustard
1 tsp dried tarragon, or
 2 bay leaves

For the topping:
Outer leaves of a large white
 cabbage
1 small cauliflower, broken
 into florets
2 large leeks, diced into
 ¼-¾ inch pieces (discard
 green ends)
2 oz Parmesan, grated
1-2 tsp paprika

Preheat the oven to 350°F. Gently fry the onions in 1 tbsp of the oil in a deep metal pie pan on the stove top—a nice trick for saving washing-up from Jamie Oliver (or use a saucepan and transfer the contents to the dish later).

When the onions have softened, add the chicken and cook until it is slightly browned, then stir in the mushrooms and nutmeg. Fry gently for a few more minutes. Scatter the cornstarch over the onions and chicken and mix it into the juices. Then pour in the chicken stock and the crème fraîche along with the mustard, tarragon, and some seasoning. Stir and simmer for a few minutes.

Meanwhile, prepare the topping by cutting each cabbage leaf in half with a sharp knife and removing the tough central stalk, then place the leaves on top of the chicken and mushroom sauce, slightly overlapping so it cooks without drying out. Mix the cauliflower and leeks in a bowl with the remaining 1 tbsp oil and season well. Spread this mixture over the layer of cabbage, scatter the Parmesan and then the paprika on top, and bake the pie for about 30 minutes, checking after about 20 minutes. Serve with green vegetables.

Tip: chicken thighs tend to have more flavor and are also cheaper than breasts.

- **CALORIES** 250
- PROTEIN 26G
- FAT 12G
- FIBER 3G
- CARBS 9G

Low-carb lamb hotpot

A classic Lancashire hotpot topped with butternut squash. This benefits from several hours of cooking so the meat melts in your mouth.

Serves 4

2 tbsp olive oil
14 oz lamb, diced
2 onions, chopped
½ tsp dried thyme
Sprig of rosemary
4 carrots, cut into batons
  (short sticks)
2 tsp cornstarch
1 tbsp Worcestershire sauce
2 cups lamb or chicken
  stock
½ tsp black peppercorns
1 butternut squash, peeled,
  halved, and sliced into
  1½-2 inch semicircles
2 oz Parmesan, grated

Preheat the oven to 325°F. Heat 1 tbsp of the oil in a medium heavy casserole dish with a lid. Add the lamb and, when it is starting to brown, stir in the onions and cook gently for a few minutes. Add the thyme, rosemary, and carrots and mix the cornstarch into the juices. Pour in the Worcestershire sauce and enough stock to cover the meat, along with the peppercorns. Stir well, cover the dish, and place it in the oven.

After about an hour, check that it has not dried out and if necessary add water. Then cover the surface with an overlapping layer of butternut squash slices. Drizzle with the remaining 1 tbsp oil, replace the lid, and return it to the oven.

After half an hour, check once again that it is not drying out (you may need to add ½ cup or so of water—if so, pour this in around the edges so the top doesn't get soggy). Then scatter the Parmesan on the surface, and cook the hotpot for another hour, until the top is golden brown. Serve with dark green vegetables such as cavolo nero or kale.

Tip: you can use celeriac (celery root) instead of butternut squash if you prefer.

- **CALORIES** 380
- PROTEIN 27G
- FAT 20G
- FIBER 5G
- CARBS 23G

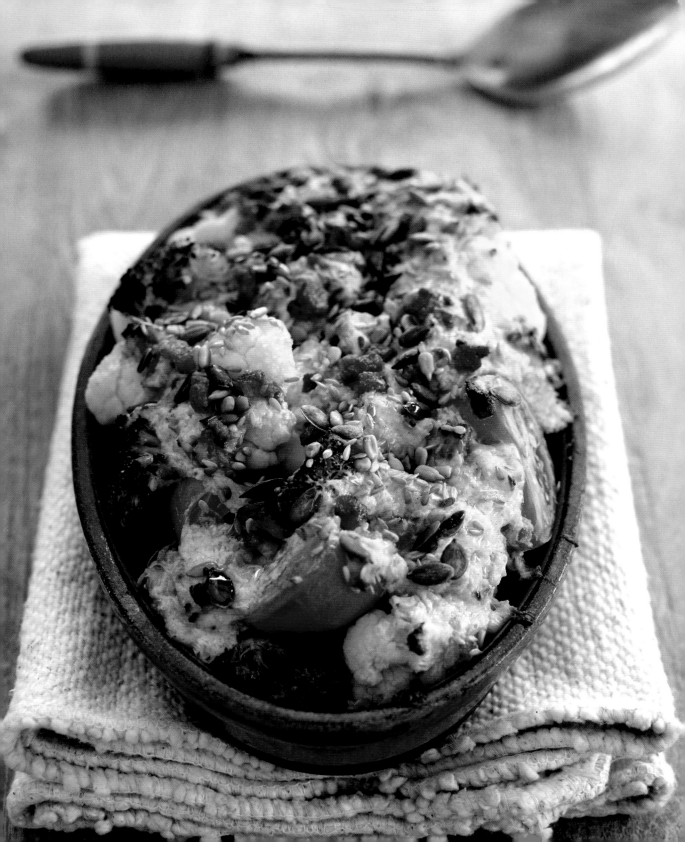

Pancetta, broccoli, and tomato gratin

Serves 4

1 head each cauliflower and
    broccoli
4 oz pancetta
Drizzle of olive oil
4 oz cream cheese
½ cup sour cream
2 oz Cheddar, grated
1 tsp mustard
2 spring onions, finely
    chopped
½ tsp cayenne pepper
2 large tomatoes, sliced
3 tbsp Parmesan, grated
3 tbsp mixed seeds

Preheat the oven to 350°F. Cut the cauliflower and
broccoli into small florets and steam them until they
are tender but still crisp, 4 to 5 minutes. Drain them
well and place them in a greased shallow baking dish.

Meanwhile, fry the pancetta in a drizzle of oil. In a
bowl, mix the cream cheese, sour cream, Cheddar,
mustard, spring onions, and cayenne and season well
with salt and pepper. Spread this mixture over the
cauliflower and broccoli as evenly as possible. Lay
the tomatoes on top of the vegetables and sprinkle
the Parmesan and seeds over the surface. Bake for
20 minutes, or until the topping is golden brown and
bubbling.

- **CALORIES** 340
- PROTEIN 22G
- FAT 23G
- FIBER 4G
- CARBS 10G

Baked fish and chorizo parcels

Serves 2

1 tbsp olive oil, plus extra
 for drizzling
1 fennel bulb, cut into
 strips
1 chorizo sausage, diced
2 thick cod steaks
2 oz cherry tomatoes, each
 pierced with a sharp knife
Handful of basil leaves
2 tbsp cider vinegar

Preheat the oven to 375°F. Heat the oil in a pan and fry the fennel and chorizo for 3 to 4 minutes.

Take 2 square sheets of aluminum foil and pile half the fennel mixture in the middle of each one. Place the cod on top, drizzle it with oil, and season well with salt and pepper. Then add the tomatoes and basil, sprinkle on the vinegar, and scrunch up the foil tightly to make a well-sealed but loose parcel. Bake the parcels for about 15 minutes and serve with salad or steamed green beans.

Tip: you could use anchovies instead of chorizo. Drape 2 to 3 fillets over each piece of cod before you put it in the oven.

- **CALORIES** 270
- PROTEIN 33G
- FAT 15G
- FIBER 1G
- CARBS 2G

Ham steak with red cabbage

The rich, sweet-tasting red cabbage works really well with the salty meat.

Serves 2

3 tbsp olive oil
1 onion, diced
½ small red cabbage, outer
 leaves removed, quartered,
 cored, and finely sliced
⅔ cup vegetable stock
4 tbsp balsamic vinegar
2 tart apples (such
 as Braeburn, Cox, or
 Granny Smith), diced into
 ¾ inch pieces
½ tsp cumin seeds, or
 ¼ tsp ground allspice
2 ham steaks, trimmed
 of fat, or 2 pork chops
1 tbsp crème fraîche
Handful of parsley or chives

Preheat the oven to 325°F. On low heat, gently cook the onion in 2 tbsp of the oil in an ovenproof casserole until it starts to caramelize. Then add the cabbage and continue to cook for a few more minutes. Add the stock, vinegar, apples, cumin seeds, and a pinch of salt and freshly ground black pepper. Cover and cook in the oven for 1 hour, stirring occasionally and adding a little water if required.

Heat the remaining 1 tbsp oil in a frying pan and fry the ham steaks on both sides. Season them with black pepper. Serve with roasted cauliflower (see page 165). Put a dollop of crème fraîche on top of the cabbage mixture and garnish with parsley.

- **CALORIES** 420
- PROTEIN 19G
- FAT 31G
- FIBER 4G
- CARBS 16G

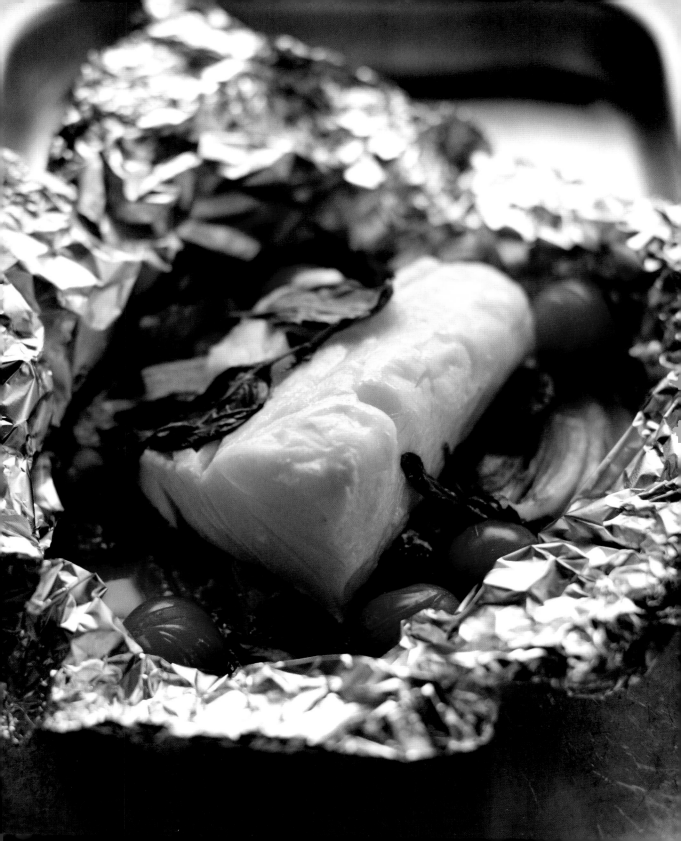

Lazy chicken and spicy lentils

This delicious dish, originally from the Caribbean, is super-easy to prepare. We have replaced the rice with lentils and love their slightly chewy, nutty taste.

Serves 4

Juice of 2 limes
3 garlic cloves, crushed
1 tsp red pepper flakes
1 tsp dried thyme
4 chicken thighs with skin (ideally boneless)
2 tbsp light olive oil
1 onion, chopped
7 oz white or cremini mushrooms, chopped
5 oz dried green lentils (or a (14-oz) can green lentils, rinsed and drained to add later)
¾ cup chicken stock (reduce to ½ cup if using canned lentils)

Combine the lime juice, garlic, red pepper flakes, and thyme in a bowl to make a marinade. Season it with pepper and salt and toss the chicken in it. Cover the bowl and leave it at room temperature for 2 hours, or in the fridge overnight.

Preheat the oven to 350°F. Then brown the chicken on both sides in 1 tbsp of the oil in a large frying pan. Scatter the onion and mushrooms over the base of a deep ovenproof dish. Add the dried lentils, place the chicken pieces on top skin side up, and drizzle with the remaining 1 tbsp oil. Pour ¾ cup stock in the bowl containing the remaining marinade juices and pour it over the chicken and vegetables. Cover the dish and place it in the oven.

After 20 minutes check it and add more stock (or some water) if it's looking dry. Cook for about 20 minutes more with the lid off (add the canned lentils at this stage, if using). Serve with green vegetables or a salad.

- **CALORIES** 460
- PROTEIN 52G
- FAT 29G
- FIBER 10G
- CARBS 52G

Michael's easy roast chicken with garlic and thyme

Roasts probably don't come to mind when you think about diet food. But a roast without the starchy potatoes or parsnips can be just that.

Serves 6

3-4 garlic cloves
Large pat of butter
2 tsp dried thyme or tarragon (sprigs of fresh even better)
1 large free-range chicken
1 lemon
1 onion, halved
14 oz whole baby carrots or carrots cut into batons (short sticks)
1 large cauliflower, broken into florets
1 tbsp olive oil
14 oz green vegetables

For the gravy:
1 tbsp cornstarch
1¼ cups hot water
1 chicken stock cube
½ tbsp soy sauce

Preheat the oven to 400°F. Mash the garlic with the butter and thyme in a small bowl. Place the chicken in a large roasting pan. Cut a few holes in the skin over the breasts and thighs, and push blobs of the garlic butter under it. Also smear some over the rest of the chicken skin and season well.

Squeeze the lemon juice over the whole chicken, rubbing it in, and put the rind inside the cavity. Add the onion to the pan cut sides down. Roast the chicken in the oven, allowing 20 minutes per pound plus 20 minutes extra. Baste it every 15 to 20 minutes. Add the carrots to the roasting pan about 40 minutes before the end of cooking time.

Place the cauliflower florets on a separate roasting pan. Season them, drizzle over the oil, and bake at the top of the oven for about 25 minutes. Also prepare the green vegetables, such as green beans, so they are ready to boil or steam while you make the gravy.

When the chicken is cooked, remove it to a carving board and let it rest. The onion can be eaten or discarded if charred. Stir the cornstarch into the oils and juices in the roasting pan, before adding 1¼ cups water, the stock cube, and the soy sauce, and continue to stir over a gentle heat until the gravy has thickened. Pour it into a warmed pitcher when you are ready to serve.

Tips: the onion in the baking pan caramelizes and produces sweet, tangy juices for a perfect gravy. Use any leftover chicken in a soup, a stir-fry, or bulgur wheat risotto (see page 129).

- **CALORIES** 260
- PROTEIN 28G
- FAT 15G
- FIBER 4G
- CARBS 17G

Vegetable Sides

We all need to eat more vegetables, whether we are on the Blood Sugar Diet or not. And you will find that on 800 calories a day they become a lifeline—filling you up and providing vital flavor, texture, and crunch. To help you reap the benefits of their huge range of health-promoting nutrients, we suggest you aim to fill half your plate at any main meal with non-starchy vegetables. These will give you a slow-release form of energy with little impact on blood sugars.

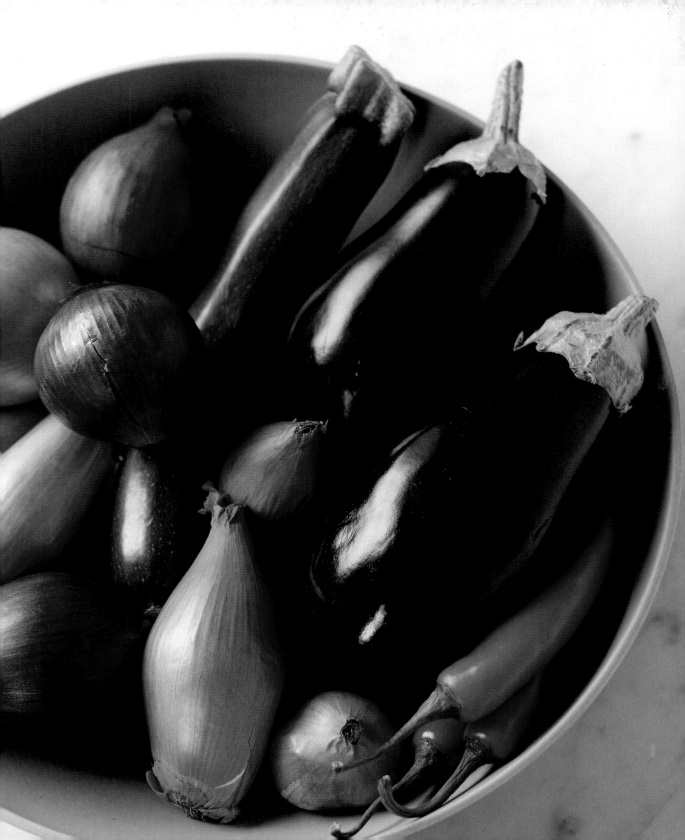

Simple salads

These make excellent side salads, but you can also add extras such as cheese, nuts, seeds, tofu, or smoked fish to turn them into a meal in themselves.

Mixed leaf salad with arugula and shaved Parmesan

You can't go wrong with this Mediterranean classic, which takes only a few minutes to prepare and goes with almost anything.

Serves 2

1 (12-oz) bag arugula
  or mixed salad leaves
1 tbsp olive oil
½ tbsp balsamic vinegar
1 oz Parmesan, shaved

Place the arugula in the bowl, drizzle over the oil and vinegar with a pinch of salt and some freshly ground black pepper, then scatter the Parmesan on top.

- CALORIES 120
- PROTEIN 7G
- FAT 10G
- FIBER 1G
- CARBS 0G

Crunchy red coleslaw

This colorful crunchy coleslaw goes particularly well with cold meats.

Serves 4

½ small red cabbage, very
  finely sliced
1 fennel bulb, finely sliced
1 small red onion, finely
  sliced
1 carrot, grated
2 tbsp pomegranate seeds,
  or 1 small red apple,
  grated
2 tbsp each mayonnaise
  and Greek yogurt,
  blended together
1 tbsp chopped walnuts,
  toasted, or 2 tsp chia
  seeds

Mix the cabbage, fennel, onion, carrot, pomegranate seeds in a bowl, stir in the mayo and yogurt dressing with a pinch of salt and some freshly ground black pepper, and scatter the nuts on top.

- CALORIES 120
- PROTEIN 3G
- FAT 9G
- FIBER 3G
- CARBS 7G

Tabbouleh with pine nuts

As with traditional tabbouleh recipes, relatively little bulgur wheat is used; it's really more of a parsley salad, which makes it an even less carb-rich addition to a meal.

Serves 4

¼ cup bulgur wheat
3 oz parsley, coarsely
  chopped
1 oz mint leaves, coarsely
  chopped
2 oz tomatoes, seeded
  and finely diced
2 oz cucumber, seeded
  and finely diced
1 spring onion, finely sliced,
  or 1 tbsp red onion
¼ cup pine nuts, toasted
  and coarsely chopped
Handful of pomegranate
  seeds or raisins

For the dressing:
1 garlic clove, crushed
2 tbsp lemon juice
3 tbsp olive oil
1 tsp cumin seeds
½ tsp ground cinnamon
½ tsp cayenne pepper

Put the bulgur wheat in a small saucepan and cover it with ¼ to ½ inch of water. Bring it to a boil, then reduce the heat and simmer for 10 minutes, adding a splash more water if necessary. Turn off the heat and let it steam, covered, for another 10 to 15 minutes.

Meanwhile, make the dressing by whisking the garlic, lemon juice, oil, cumin seeds, cinnamon, and cayenne in a small bowl with some salt and freshly ground black pepper.

Mix the mint, tomatoes, cucumber, spring onion, and pine nuts together in a bowl. When the bulgur wheat has cooled, add it to the salad and stir in the dressing before scattering over the pomegranate seeds.

Tip: toasting pine nuts brings out the flavor—simply put them in a dry frying pan over a medium to high heat, shaking and stirring intermittently for a few minutes until they are golden brown.

- **CALORIES** 150
- PROTEIN 4G
- FAT 9G
- FIBER 2G
- CARBS 13G

Broccoli and asparagus salad

The creamy, tangy buttermilk dressing here really brings this salad to life. Buttermilk contains healthy live bacteria which are good for your gut, while the broccoli is rich in antioxidants which mop up damaging free radicals.

Serves 4

1 head broccoli
1 large bunch asparagus
  (about 12 stems)
Buttermilk dressing (see
  page 176)
1 tbsp sliced almonds

Break the broccoli into small florets and cut the asparagus into 1½ to 1¾ inch lengths. If the asparagus is thick, slice it lengthwise first. Put the vegetables in a large bowl and drizzle the buttermilk dressing over. Toast the almonds in a small dry frying pan for 1 to 2 minutes (watch closely as they burn quickly), then scatter them over the salad.

Tip: if you prefer your broccoli and asparagus a bit softer you can sear it briefly in a frying pan or under the broiler first.

- **CALORIES** 60
- PROTEIN 5G
- FAT 4G
- FIBER 3G
- CARBS 2G

Spiced purple vegetables

Delicious hot or cold, this dish livens up almost any meal. There is evidence of lots of health benefits from eating beets, including lowering blood pressure, reducing the risk of heart disease and dementia, and improving muscle aches after exercise.

Serves 4

2 medium beets, peeled
1 large red onion, sliced
½ small red cabbage, cored
  and finely sliced
3 tbsp balsamic or cider
  vinegar
½ tsp cumin seeds
½ tsp coriander seeds
½ tsp red chile, seeded
  and finely diced, or
  ½ tsp red pepper flakes

Chop the beets into ¾-inch cubes and place them in a colander. Then add layers of onion and cabbage, sprinkling salt between each as you go. Leave the colander over a bowl to drain for about 20 minutes.

Preheat the oven to 325°C. Rinse and drain the salted vegetables over the sink. Then place all the vegetables in a baking dish, pour over the vinegar, scatter the spices and mix together along with a pinch salt and freshly ground black pepper on top. Cover the dish with foil and bake for 30 minutes, turning the vegetables once. Serve hot or cold.

- **CALORIES** 40
- PROTEIN 2G
- FAT 0G
- FIBER 3G
- CARBS 9G

Pickled cabbage (kimchi)

It is now recognized that pickling food in vinegar provides health benefits, lowering blood sugars and boosting your gut bacteria.

Makes 2 portions

½ small white cabbage or Chinese cabbage, cored and outer leaves removed
2 garlic cloves, finely chopped
¾ inch fresh ginger, finely chopped or grated
1 tbsp mirin or cider vinegar
1 tbsp Thai fish sauce, or soy sauce
2 tsp sweet chili sauce (see page 175), or 1-2 tsp red pepper flakes and 1 tsp hoisin plum sauce
2 spring onions, finely chopped
1 tsp maple syrup or honey
¼ tsp salt

Finely slice the cabbage and steam or microwave it for 2 minutes. Then place it in a large jar with a lid or in a covered bowl. Meanwhile, make the marinade by mixing the garlic, ginger, mirin, fish sauce, chili sauce, spring onions, maple syrup, and salt in a bowl. Pour the marinade over the cabbage, mix it well and ideally leave it for up to 6 hours, but for a minimum of 30 minutes, stirring occasionally.

- **CALORIES** 80
- PROTEIN 4G
- FAT 1G
- FIBER 3G
- CARBS 14G

Rainbow salad

I encourage my patients to eat not only more vegetables, but also different colored vegetables. As well as making food look more enticing, the different colors represent different phytochemicals, substances which plants produce to protect themselves against bacteria, viruses, and so on, and which are also good for our health.

Serves 2

2 large handfuls of
  watercress
1 carrot, grated
1 pickled beet, diced
1 yellow bell pepper,
  seeded and cut
  into strips
8 cherry tomatoes, halved
4 radishes, finely sliced
Handful of blueberries

Put all the salad ingredients in a large bowl and toss them in French vinaigrette (see page 173).

Tip: most supermarkets sell pickled beets.

- **CALORIES** 120
- PROTEIN 3G
- FAT 1G
- FIBER 4G
- CARBS 11G

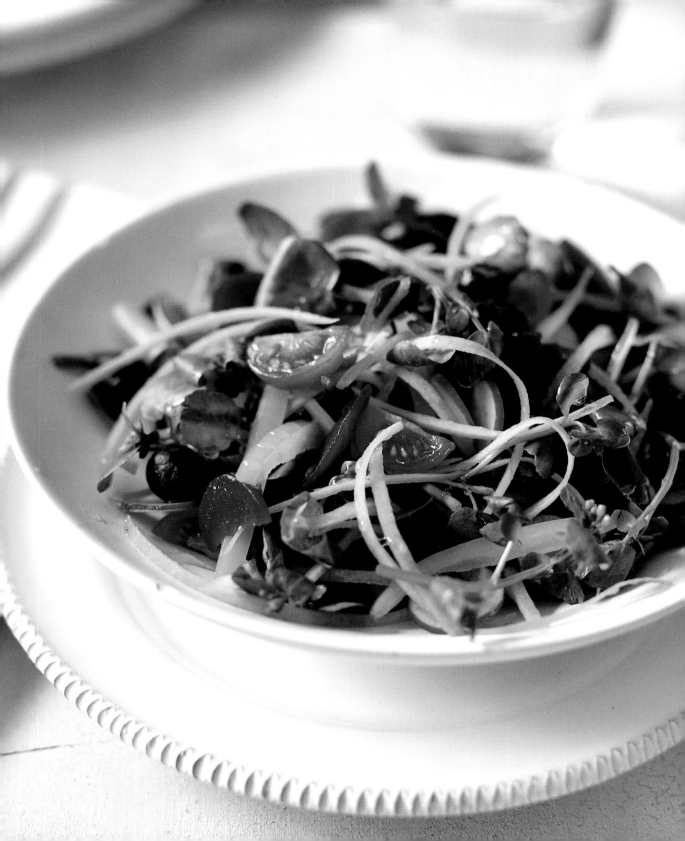

Cooked vegetable sides

Roasted garlicky eggplant mash

This dish is a faster and easier version of the Middle Eastern classic baba ganoush in which eggplants are charred under the broiler, producing a wonderful smoky flavor. It works brilliantly as a side dish or it can be eaten as a dip with vegetable sticks, as a lighter alternative to hummus.

Serves 4

2 eggplants
2 tbsp olive oil
1 onion, finely diced
2 garlic cloves, crushed
½ tbsp balsamic vinegar
½ tsp chile, seeded and
* finely diced, or ½ tsp*
* red pepper flakes (to taste)*
Handful of parsley, chopped
1 tbsp pomegranate
* seeds (optional)*

There are several ways to roast the eggplants. We do it in our old iron wok, with the heat high and the lid on. It takes about 5 minutes and there's no mess. Place the eggplants in the hot dry wok, stalks still on, and cover. To get the flavor, the skin has to burn so allow it to thicken and char before you turn it. You don't need to char it all but aim to do at least half.

Meanwhile, heat the oil in a medium saucepan with a lid and gently cook the onions for about 5 minutes, then stir in the garlic.

When the eggplants are sufficiently charred, transfer them to a plate and allow them to cool a bit. Or if you're in a hurry, keep a glass of cold water nearby to cool your fingers as you prepare them. Chop off the stalks and peel the skin, then dice the flesh and add it to the pan. Stir in the vinegar and chile.

Cook gently for 10 to 15 minutes, with the lid on, stirring occasionally. Add 1 tbsp of water if it is drying out to maintain a thick creamy texture. Season and serve with parsley and pomegranate seeds, if using, scattered over.

Tips: there are other ways to char the eggplant skin. You can hold it with tongs directly over a hot flame on a gas burner (but this can be messy, when the skin bursts and juice drips everywhere); or place it under a hot broiler, piercing the skin first, and turning it several times.

- **CALORIES** 90
- PROTEIN 1G
- FAT 7G
- FIBER 2G
- CARBS 5G

Cauliflower 2 ways

Having barely eaten cauliflower since school days, we have rediscovered it in a big way. When baked it has a slightly nutty taste, and it makes an ideal replacement for potatoes.

1. Simple roasted cauliflower

Serves 2

1 large cauliflower, broken
  into florets
1 tbsp olive oil
1 tbsp Parmesan, grated

Preheat the oven to 350°F. Spread the cauliflower over a baking sheet, season it with salt and freshly ground black pepper, drizzle with the oil, and sprinkle with the Parmesan. Roast it for about 20 minutes, turning it halfway through. It is cooked when it has started to soften but is still firm.

• **CALORIES** 130
• PROTEIN 9G
• FAT 8G
• FIBER 4G
• CARBS 6G

2. Spicy roasted cauliflower

Serves 2

2 tbsp coconut, olive,
  or rapeseed oil
Juice of 1 lemon
3 garlic cloves, peeled
  and halved
¼ inch fresh ginger, grated
3 tsp garam masala
1 tsp red chile, seeded
  and finely diced, or
  1 tsp red pepper flakes
1 large cauliflower, broken
  into florets
1 tbsp sliced almond

Preheat the oven to 350°F. Mix the oil, lemon juice, garlic, ginger, garam masala, and chile in a large bowl. Add the cauliflower florets, season, and mix well.

Spread the cauliflower on a baking sheet and roast for about 20 minutes, turning it halfway through. The cauliflower should be al dente. Sprinkle over the almonds 5 minutes before removing the dish from the oven.

Tip: you can add other vegetables such as broccoli florets or asparagus.

• **CALORIES** 220
• PROTEIN 8G
• FAT 18G
• FIBER 4G
• CARBS 6G

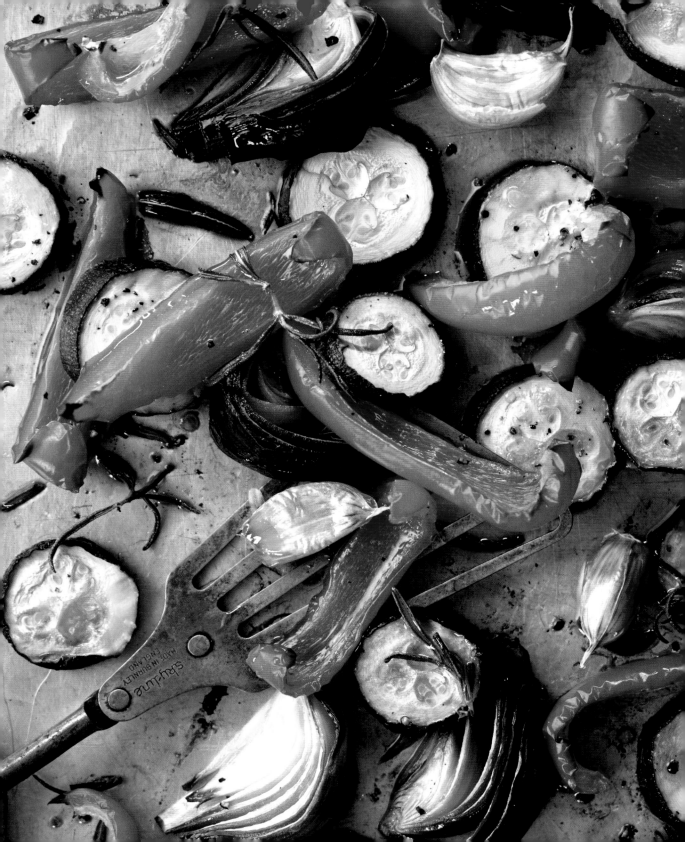

Roasted Mediterranean vegetables

Serves 4

3 garlic cloves, crushed
3 tbsp olive oil
1 red and 1 yellow bell
    pepper, seeded and
    quartered
1 eggplant, diced
1 zucchini, sliced or diced
1 fennel bulb, sliced
3 tomatoes, quartered
½ red onion, sliced
Sprigs of thyme and
    rosemary

Preheat the oven to 400°F. In a bowl, mix the garlic with the oil and season with salt and black pepper (and a pinch of red pepper flakes, if you wish). Arrange the eggplant, zucchini, fennel, tomatoes, and onion in a roasting pan, scatter over the thyme and rosemary and drizzle with the flavored oil. Roast for 30 to 40 minutes, turning once after about 15 minutes.

Tip: when roasting vegetables, make sure you spread them out well on the baking sheet or dish so that they don't get soggy.

- **CALORIES** 130
- PROTEIN 3G
- FAT 9G
- FIBER 5G
- CARBS 12G

Creamed spinach

Some people find cooked spinach bitter—the crème fraîche counteracts this beautifully.

Serves 2

7 oz fresh spinach
Pat of butter, or ½ tbsp
    olive oil
2 heaping tbsp crème
    fraîche
½ tsp ground nutmeg

If you are using fresh spinach you just need to heat it in a saucepan with the oil for 2 to 3 minutes, or until it wilts. Thawing frozen spinach in a saucepan will take a few minutes longer. Drain it well and transfer it to a dish. Stir in the crème fraîche, nutmeg, and plenty of seasoning.

Tip: make double quantities as it freezes really well.

- **CALORIES** 160
- PROTEIN 3G
- FAT 15G
- FIBER 2G
- CARBS 2G

Peas and edamame with yogurt and lime dressing

Serves 2

¼ cup frozen peas
¼ cup frozen edamame
    beans
2 tbsp crème fraîche
Handful of dill, chopped
Handful of chives, chopped
Squeeze of lime juice

Put the peas and edamame in a pan of boiling water and simmer for 3 to 4 minutes, then drain them and allow to cool. In a bowl, mix the crème fraîche with the dill, chives, lime juice, and some seasoning, and stir in the peas and beans.

- **CALORIES** 230
- PROTEIN 5G
- FAT 21G
- FIBER 3G
- CARBS 6G

6 simple ways to get your greens

1. Broccoli with garlic and anchovy

Broccoli contains generous amounts of antioxidant phytochemicals and the more bitter it tastes, the better it is for your health. Unfortunately, to increase sales, most modern supermarket vegetables have had the bitterness bred out of them. This dish is so tasty and nutritious that it could be a meal in itself.

Serves 4

1 tbsp olive oil
1 garlic clove, crushed or chopped
2 sprigs rosemary
½ tsp red chile, seeded and finely diced, or ½ tsp red pepper flakes (optional)
3 anchovies from a jar, chopped
7 oz tenderstem broccoli, long stems included
Squeeze of lemon
1 tbsp pine nuts or sliced almonds, toasted (optional)

In a large pan, heat the oil and sauté the garlic, rosemary, and chile, if using, for a few minutes. Remove the rosemary, add the anchovies and simmer for another 3 to 5 minutes, crushing the anchovies into a paste with a wooden spoon as they cook.

Boil, steam, or microwave the broccoli for just a couple of minutes, so it retains a slight crunch. Drain the broccoli and stir it into the anchovy mixture. Add a generous squeeze of lemon, season, and scatter over the toasted nuts or seeds, if using, before serving.

- **CALORIES** 90
- PROTEIN 5G
- FAT 8G
- FIBER 3G
- CARBS 2G

2. Swiss chard stir-fried with garlic

So simple and so good. And it goes with almost anything. Choose fresh seasonal alternatives if possible—kale, spring greens, or cabbage also work well.

Serves 2

1 tbsp olive or rapeseed oil
1 garlic clove, crushed or sliced
7 oz Swiss chard, sliced

Place a frying pan or wok over high heat, add the oil, and fry the garlic for a minute before adding the chard. Turn down the heat to medium, add 1 tbsp of warm water and some seasoning, and cook for 2 to 3 minutes, tossing it frequently, until it is tender but still crisp. Transfer immediately to a dish and serve.

- **CALORIES** 76
- PROTEIN 3G
- FAT 6G
- FIBER 2G
- CARBS 2G

3. Cabbage stir-fried Chinese style

Serves 2

1 tbsp coconut or rapeseed oil
¼ inch fresh ginger, finely chopped
1 garlic clove, chopped (optional)
½ small cabbage, cored and leaves finely diced
5 oz bean sprouts
1 tbsp soy sauce
1 tsp sesame oil (optional)

Place a frying pan or wok over high heat, add the coconut oil, and fry the ginger and garlic, if using, for a minute before adding the cabbage. Turn down the heat to medium, add 1 tbsp of warm water, and cook the cabbage for 2 minutes, tossing it frequently, until it is tender but still crisp.

Add the bean sprouts and sauté them gently for a minute, before stirring in the soy sauce and sesame oil, if using. Transfer the vegetables immediately to a dish, season, and serve.

- **CALORIES** 80
- PROTEIN 3G
- FAT 6G
- FIBER 2G
- CARBS 2G

4. Bok choy with oyster sauce

This makes an ideal accompaniment to Chinese pork meatballs (see page 85).

Serves 2

1 tbsp coconut or rapeseed oil
7 oz bok choy or other fresh greens
1 tbsp oyster sauce
1 tsp sesame oil (optional)

Place a frying pan or wok over high heat, add the coconut oil, and then the bok choy. Turn down the heat to medium, add 1 tbsp of warm water, and cook for 2 minutes, tossing them frequently. Then stir in the oyster sauce and drizzle with the sesame oil, if using. The bok choy is done when it is tender but still crisp. Transfer to a dish and serve immediately.

- **CALORIES** 170
- PROTEIN 4G
- FAT 12G
- FIBER 5G
- CARBS 11G

5. Spring greens with garlic and cannellini beans

Beans make up an important part of the Mediterranean-style diet and work really well slipped into a dish to add taste and texture. They also make it significantly more filling.

Serves 2

1 tbsp olive oil
1 garlic clove, crushed
½ tsp red pepper flakes
½ tsp dried thyme
  or oregano
8 cherry tomatoes, halved
4 oz canned cannellini
  beans, rinsed and drained
7 oz spring greens, finely
  sliced, or mature spinach
Squeeze of lemon

Heat the oil in a saucepan with a lid and add the garlic, red pepper flakes, and thyme, followed by the tomatoes, beans, and greens. Then add ½ tbsp of water and a generous squeeze of lemon and some seasoning.

Stir and simmer with the lid on until the greens are cooked, 2 to 3 minutes, or until just wilted. Transfer them to a dish and serve.

- **CALORIES** 130
- PROTEIN 7G
- FAT 7G
- FIBER 6G
- CARBS 12G

6. Green beans with soy sauce and sesame seeds

An adaptation of a lovely Japanese recipe given to us by chef Akemi Yokoyama. Delicious, quick, and easy.

Serves 2

7 oz haricots verts, cut in
  half, or snow peas
2 tbsp white sesame seeds
1 tbsp soy sauce
1 tsp sesame oil
1 tsp hoisin plum sauce, or
  ½ tsp maple syrup

Bring a pan of water to a boil and add the beans with a pinch of salt. Cook them for 3 minutes (less for snow peas) over medium heat, or until they are just tender. Then run them under cold water in a sieve, drain them, and set aside.

Dry-roast the sesame seeds in a frying pan or wok over low heat, stirring all the time. Remove them as soon as they start to brown (after about 1 minute) and immediately transfer them to a dish to stop them from burning.

Using the same pan, turn up the heat to medium and throw in the beans with the oil, then add the soy sauce and plum sauce. Sauté for 1 minute, and season to taste. Serve immediately.

- **CALORIES** 120
- PROTEIN 6G
- FAT 9G
- FIBER 3G
- CARBS 6G

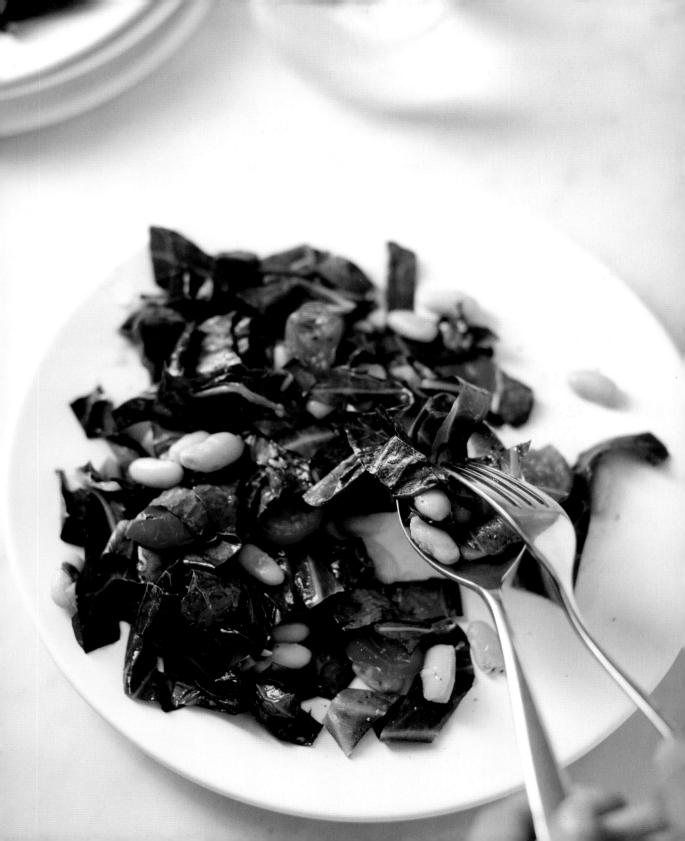

Dressings

Some dressings require a small amount of sugar or honey to counteract the vinegar or lemon. Although this goes somewhat against the principles of the Blood Sugar Diet, if it helps you enjoy and eat more vegetables then it is a compromise worth making. In the scheme of things, half a teaspoon of maple syrup or honey in a dressing is insignificant as part of a meal.

Mayo 4 ways

It's wonderful to have mayonnaise back on the menu, now that we are being encouraged to eat more healthy fats with our food. You can of course make your own, but a good-quality store-bought mayo works well, particularly if you add different flavors to it. Remember that full-fat is better for you and tastes better, too, though it is also high in calories, so watch the quantities.

All the following make 2 portions

1. Light lemon mayo

Perfect with asparagus tips.

Zest of 1 lemon
1 tbsp full-fat mayonnaise
1 tbsp full-fat Greek yogurt

Beat the lemon zest, mayonnaise, and yogurt together and adjust the seasoning.

- **CALORIES** 75
- PROTEIN 2G
- FAT 8G
- FIBER 0G
- CARBS 1G

2. Garlic mayo

2 tbsp full-fat mayonnaise
1 tbsp full-fat Greek yogurt
½ garlic clove, crushed
1 tbsp chives or dill, chopped (optional)

Beat the mayonnaise, yogurt, garlic, and chives, if using, together and adjust the seasoning.

- **CALORIES** 130
- PROTEIN 1G
- FAT 14G
- FIBER 0G
- CARBS 1G

3. Anchovy mayo

1 tbsp full-fat mayonnaise
1 tbsp olive oil
1 tbsp lime or lemon juice
6 anchovies from a jar or
  can, finely chopped
1 tbsp minced rosemary
  leaves

Mix together the mayo, oil, and lime juice to form a creamy texture, add the anchovies and rosemary with some freshly ground black pepper and mix energetically to infuse the flavors.

- **CALORIES 150**
- PROTEIN 2G
- FAT 16
- FIBER 0G
- CARBS 0G

4. Chili mayo

Great as a dip or with seafood. Worth making the sweet chili sauce for this alone.

1 tbsp low-sugar sweet chili
  sauce (see page 175)
1 tbsp full-fat mayonnaise

Beat the chili sauce and mayonnaise together and adjust the seasoning.

- **CALORIES 105**
- PROTEIN 1G
- FAT 10G
- FIBER 0G
- CARBS 1G

French vinaigrette

Makes 4 portions

4 tbsp olive oil
2 tbsp lemon juice
1 tsp spicy brown, Dijon, or
  grainy mustard
¼ garlic clove, crushed
  (optional)

Beat the oil, lemon juice, mustard, and garlic together and adjust the seasoning.

- **CALORIES 100**
- PROTEIN 0G
- FAT 11G
- FIBER 0G
- CARBS 2G

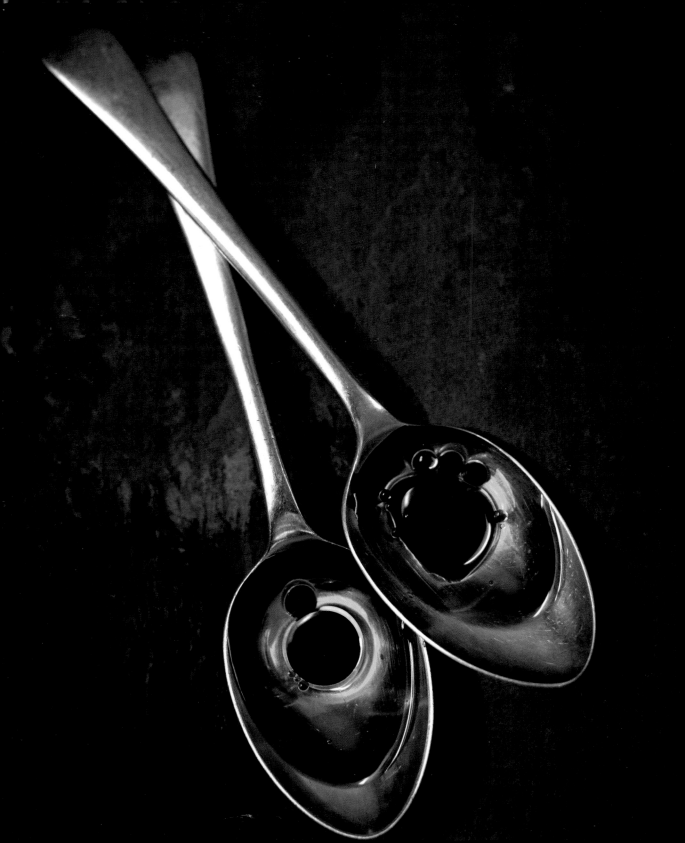

Yogurt 2 ways

Makes 2 portions

1. Yogurt and mustard dressing

2 tsp spicy brown mustard
½ tbsp olive oil
½ tbsp walnut oil
1 tbsp full-fat plain
 yogurt

- **CALORIES** 70
- PROTEIN 1G
- FAT 3G
- FIBER 0G
- CARBS 1G

Beat the mustard, oils, and yogurt and adjust the seasoning.

2. Garlic and lemon yogurt dressing

2 tbsp full-fat Greek yogurt
½ garlic clove, crushed
Zest of half a lemon
1 mint leaf, finely chopped
 (optional)

- **CALORIES** 40
- PROTEIN 2G
- FAT 3G
- FIBER 0G
- CARBS 1G

Beat the yogurt, garlic, lemon zest, and mint and adjust the seasoning.

Low-sugar sweet chili sauce

Makes 6 portions

Instead of cornstarch, this recipe uses the natural thickening properties of chia seeds, so it contains very little starchy carbohydrate. It tastes as good, is easier to make, and remarkably authentic.

1-2 red chiles, seeded
 and very finely diced
½ small red bell pepper,
 seeded and very finely
 diced
¼ inch fresh ginger, grated
1 garlic clove, crushed
1 tsp chia seeds
1 tbsp balsamic vinegar
1 tbsp mirin wine
¼ tsp salt
1 tbsp Thai fish sauce

Place the chiles, bell pepper, ginger, garlic, chia seeds, vinegar, mirin, salt, and fish sauce in a pan along with 2 tbsp of water, cover, and simmer for 4 to 5 minutes, stirring regularly (or microwave for 3 to 4 minutes). Add an extra tablespoon of water gradually if the consistency is too thick. Pour the sauce into a clean glass container with a lid and store it in the fridge.

Tip: chia seeds have an extraordinary ability to absorb fluid to form a gel, ideal for thickening a sauce. If you don't have any, stir in 1 tsp cornstarch instead.

- **CALORIES** 40
- PROTEIN 1G
- FAT 2G
- FIBER 2G
- CARBS 1G

Buttermilk dressing

The live cultured buttermilk gives this dressing a wonderful creamy, tangy taste. Fermented milk not only improves our ability to absorb nutrients but also helps restore the balance of healthy bacteria in our gut. What's more, it contains significantly fewer calories than whole milk.

Makes 4 portions

¼ cup buttermilk
¼ cup full-fat mayonnaise
1 tbsp cider vinegar
½ tsp maple syrup
  (optional)

Mix the buttermilk, mayonnaise, vinegar, and maple syrup together with a generous pinch of salt and black pepper.

- **CALORIES** 70
- PROTEIN 1G
- FAT 6G
- FIBER 0G
- CARBS 1G

Red salsa

So much nicer than the store-bought version.

Makes 2 portions

5 oz tomatoes, finely
  chopped
½ garlic clove, chopped
½ tbsp cider vinegar
2 tbsp olive oil
½ small red bell pepper,
  seeded and diced
½ tsp red chile, seeded
  and finely diced, or
  ½ tsp red pepper flakes
  (to taste)
Handful of parsley or
  cilantro, chopped

Mix the tomatoes, garlic, vinegar, oil, bell pepper, chile, and parsley together in a bowl and season with salt and black pepper.

- **CALORIES** 140
- PROTEIN 1G
- FAT 13G
- FIBER 2G
- CARBS 5G

Home-made pesto

Easy to make and bursting with flavor.

Makes 4 portions

¼ cup chopped walnuts,
  toasted
¼ cup pine nuts, toasted
2 oz basil leaves, chopped
5 tbsp olive oil
Juice of 2 lemons

Blitz the walnuts, pine nuts, basil, oil, and lemon juice in a blender or in a food processor. Season and store in a clean jar in the fridge for a few days or in the freezer.

- **CALORIES** 160
- PROTEIN 2G
- FAT 17G
- FIBER 0G
- CARBS 1G

Toppings

Scatter these on top of soups, fish, vegetables, or salads to add extra flavor.

- **Chorizo or andouille sausage:** great with white fish or scallops, or on top of soups; ½ oz sausage, very finely chopped and roasted or fried (= 60 calories)

- **Pancetta:** this adds flavor and extra protein to soup, and is delicious scattered on a bake or salad; ½ oz pancetta fried gently in a dash of olive oil until crispy and golden brown, with a crushed garlic clove for extra flavor (= 70 calories)

- **Roasted nuts and seeds:** the toasting brings out the flavors, giving them a sweet and nutty taste. Keep them in an airtight jam jar. Half a handful of sesame seeds, pine nuts, pumpkin, chia, or other seeds (either cooked in a frying pan or baked in the oven, or dry-roasted in a nonstick frying pan).

- **Diced feta** (1 oz = 80 calories) or **fried halloumi cheese** (1½ oz = 130 calories)

- **Garlic-sautéed kale:** to sprinkle on top of soups; 2 oz kale, leaves torn off and sautéed for a few minutes in 1 tsp olive oil with a crushed garlic clove (= 50 calories)

- **Sliced mushrooms:** 2 oz finely sliced mushrooms sautéed in a pat of butter with a chopped garlic clove, garnished with finely chopped parsley (= 50 calories)

Occasional Treats

This chapter is all about showing you that, even while on the Blood Sugar Diet, you can eat <u>occasional</u> treats, our thinking being that it is better to have the odd cake or dessert which is low in sugar and relatively low-carb than risk being tempted by sweet, carb-rich alternatives.

Bread is more tricky, because it is an everyday food that people generally find much harder to cut down on. The more you train yourself to do without it, the better your chances of keeping the weight off in the long term. So we recommend that while you are on the 800-calorie-a-day regime you keep your bread intake to an absolute minimum. If and when you do eat bread, make it the relatively solid and chewy kind containing unrefined whole grains and seeds, like those we have included here.

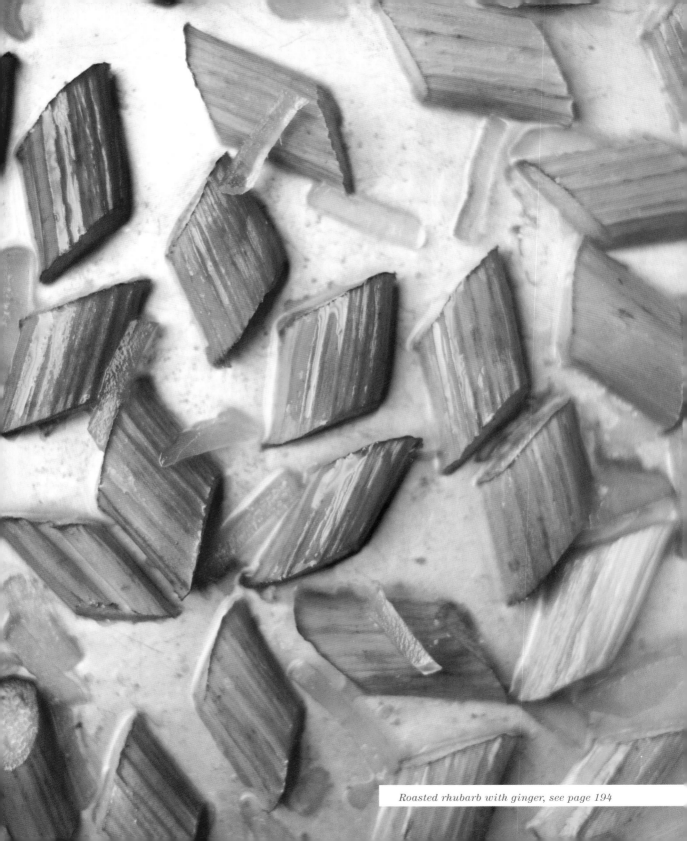

Roasted rhubarb with ginger, see page 194

Breads and flatbread

There are now so many different flours available—not just wheat and rye, but also nut varieties, such as coconut, almond, or chestnut—that making a choice can be daunting. The flours come in different degrees of "refinement," from coarsely chopped, to ground, to fully refined. This affects how much fiber remains in them and whether the healthy oils and nutrients have been removed or not. The amount of processing will also determine whether they are low or high GI and how great a sugar spike they cause.

If you are used to standard processed wheat flour you will find that nut flours behave differently when used for baking. Some absorb lots of fluid, some have a grainy texture and, to make things even more complicated, the proportions of flour to liquid required are often not quite equivalent. Stick closely to the recipes, and you will be fine!

Whole grain soda bread

According to Elizabeth David, "Everyone who cooks should know how to make a loaf of soda bread." It really is easy. It doesn't require yeast, kneading, or time to rise.

Makes 12 slices
(calories are per slice)

2¼ cups whole wheat flour
½ cup spelt flour
2 tbsp rolled oats
2 tsp baking soda
½ tsp salt
2 tbsp pumpkin seeds, plus extra for sprinkling
2 tbsp sunflower seeds, plus extra for sprinkling
3 oz walnuts, chopped
1¼ cups buttermilk
3-4 tbsp milk
1 tbsp olive oil

Preheat the oven to 450°F. Place the flours, oats, baking soda, and salt in a mixing bowl with the seeds and walnuts. Stir in the buttermilk. Mix gently to make a soft dough, adding the milk gradually. Shape the dough on a floured surface and place it in an oiled 2 lb loaf pan. Alternatively, shape it into a flattened ball and cut a cross into the surface for a more traditional shape. Scatter the rest of the seeds over the work surface and roll the loaf over them so they stick to it.

Bake the loaf for 10 minutes, then reduce the temperature to 400°F and bake for another 20 to 30 minutes, until it is golden and firm.

Tip: we suggest you slice any bread you don't eat and keep it in a bag in the freezer. Cooling the bread will also convert some of the starchy carbohydrate into more fibrous "resistant starch" which has less impact on blood sugar (note—only some of the starch!).

- **CALORIES** 210
- PROTEIN 7G
- FAT 8G
- FIBER 3G
- CARBS 29G

Seeded spelt and rye bread

Spelt or hulled wheat, cultivated since 5000 BC, is a hardier and more nutritious cousin of modern wheat and has a sweetish, slightly nutty taste. This bread, adapted from a lovely recipe by JPS Cloud on the website, is easy to make, particularly in a breadmaker. You can adjust the proportions of the flour—just note that the more rye you add, the less it rises.

Makes 12 slices
(calories are per slice)

2¾ cups stone-ground
  spelt flour
¾ cup plus 2 tbsp stone-
  ground rye flour
1½ tsp salt
2 tsp yeast
3 tbsp seeds of your choice:
  we suggest 1 tbsp poppy
  (these are small and don't
  overwhelm the bread),
  1 tbsp sunflower, and
  1 tbsp flaxseeds or
  pumpkin seeds
1¾ cups lukewarm water
2 tbsp olive oil, or 3 tbsp
  butter
1 tbsp honey

Put all the ingredients in the breadmaker and set as a "large" loaf on the whole grain cycle (takes 4 to 5 hours, depending on the breadmaker). Easy.

Or you can bake it in the oven. Put the flours, salt, yeast, and seeds in a large bowl and mix them together. Then gradually stir in the lukewarm water along with the oil and honey to form a dough. Use your hands to finish mixing it. There should be none left sticking to the bowl.

Transfer the dough to a flat surface scattered lightly with flour and knead it for 5 minutes, until it no longer feels sticky. Add more flour as needed. Oil the loaf pan and fold the dough into a shape that fits inside it, pressing it in evenly. Put it in a large plastic food bag and leave it to rise for 2 hours (until the dough no longer springs back when you press it with your finger). Then remove it from the bag and place it in an oven preheated to 400°F.

Remove the pan after 35 to 40 minutes. It should have risen and turned golden brown. Turn the bread out onto the baking tray. It should sound hollow when you tap it. If you like crisp crusts, put it back in the oven for 5 minutes more.

Tip: kneading bread should be a bit of an upper body workout as you need to repeatedly stretch the dough by pushing it away from you with the base of your hand, then fold it onto itself and repeat, for at least 5 minutes.

- **CALORIES** 180
- PROTEIN 5G
- FAT 5G
- FIBER 4G
- CARBS 30G

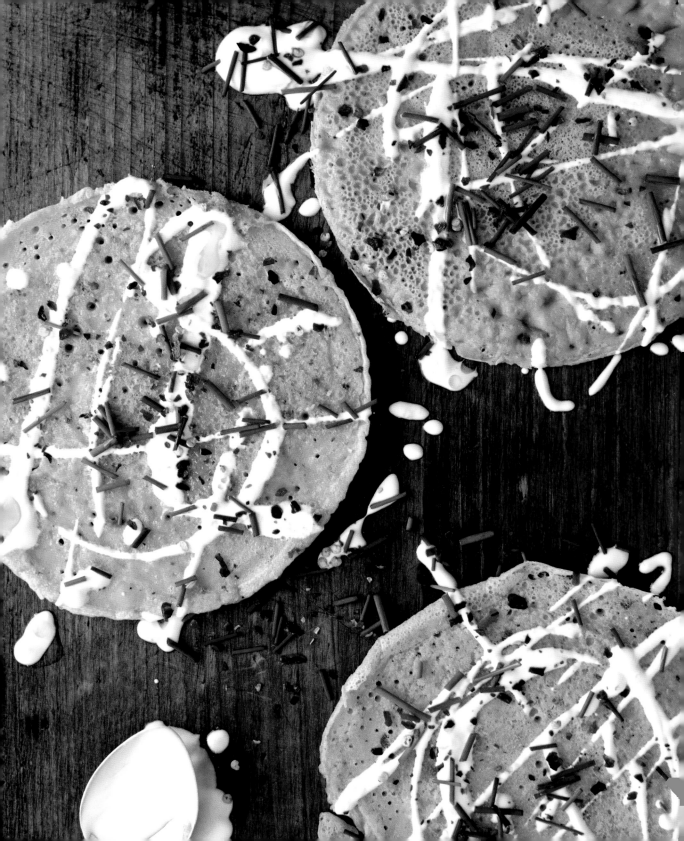

Chickpea flatbread

Many of my Asian patients with blood sugar problems tell me that they struggle to replace flatbreads or chapattis in their diet. Unfortunately, most store-bought flatbreads these days are made of highly refined wheat flour, whereas in India they are traditionally made with whole meal chickpea flour, which is relatively lower in carbohydrate and high in protein and fiber. It is also gluten-free. This is what we have used here. Chickpea flour can be found online and in most health food shops and Asian supermarkets. This is adapted from an excellent recipe posted online by Ingenue.

Makes 8

2 cups chickpea flour
(also known as gram flour
or besan)
Pinch of salt
Seasoning: we use pinches
of red pepper flakes,
pepper, and onion powder,
and either rosemary or
caraway seeds.
1 tbsp coconut or olive oil

Put the chickpea flour in a bowl and add enough water to make a thin pancake batter, whisking well as you go. Add the salt and seasoning, and then leave it to stand for 2 to 3 hours. When you are ready to use it, whisk in the oil. Put a frying pan on medium-high heat. If the pan is not nonstick, lightly brush it with oil. Swirl the batter into the pan and cook it until it is brown and crisp, turning once.

Tip: these can also be used as pizza bases, or as wraps to fill with salad, tuna, and mayonnaise or other healthy choices. They freeze well.

- **CALORIES** 110
- PROTEIN 6G
- FAT 3G
- FIBER 3G
- CARBS 16G

Desserts for now and then

Eat them slowly, in small portions—and enjoy!

Instant creamy passion fruit pudding

Incredibly easy to assemble—and looks very inviting layered in a glass.

Serves 1

2 tbsp crème fraîche or
* full-fat coconut yogurt*
1 passion fruit
Handful of berries
½ mint leaf, finely chopped
½ tsp maple syrup (optional
* and ideally skipped!)*

Put the crème fraîche in a small glass. Cut the passion fruit in half, scoop out the seeds and juice and pour them onto the crème fraîche. Scatter the berries and the mint on top and drizzle with the maple syrup, if using.

- **CALORIES** 240
- PROTEIN 2G
- FAT 24G
- FIBER 1G
- CARBS 5G

Quick chia kulfi

Inspired by a pistachio kulfi, a delightful dessert that we ate in an Indian restaurant recently, this is an easy alternative, with a similarly delicate exotic flavor and no added sugar.

Serves 2

⅔ cup coconut cream
½ oz pistachios (¾ of
* these crushed)*
1½ tsp chia seeds
Seeds from 3 cardamom
* pods*
Pinch of salt
Small handful of berries
* (optional)*

In a small pan, gently heat the coconut cream, crushed pistachios, chia and cardamom seeds. Add the salt and simmer for about 5 minutes. Pour the mixture into 2 small bowls or ramekins and place them in the fridge for 1 to 2 hours to set. Scatter the remaining pistachios and the berries, if using, over the top.

Tip: to seed the cardamom, crush the pod gently with the flat of a knife, then remove the seeds.

- **CALORIES** 360
- PROTEIN 6G
- FAT 36G
- FIBER 1G
- CARBS 6G

Orange and pistachio cupcakes

These have an exotic taste, reminiscent of a North African sweet treat, but without the syrup. They are very low-carb and contain a satisfying amount of protein.

Makes 6
(calories are per cake)

1 large egg
2 tbsp coconut oil or butter, melted
Zest and juice of 1 orange
5 large pitted dates, very finely chopped
½ cup ground almonds
1 tsp baking powder
Seeds from 3 cardamom pods
1 oz pistachios, coarsely crushed
6 good-size raspberries
¼ tsp salt

Preheat the oven to 325°F. Mix the egg, oil, and orange zest and juice with the dates and blitz them in a blender or in a food processor (or with a fork). Then stir in the almonds, baking powder, and cardamom seeds along with half of the pistachios. Mix everything vigorously. Spoon the mixture into 6 paper cupcake cases and set them aside for a few minutes to let the baking powder act. Press a raspberry into the middle of each cupcake and scatter the remaining pistachios on top. Bake the cakes for about 15 minutes. They are done when they are golden brown and springy to the touch.

- **CALORIES** 360
- PROTEIN 10G
- FAT 25G
- FIBER 4G
- CARBS 25G

Almond pancakes with cherries

Serves 4

2 oz cherries, halved and
   pitted
2 eggs
1 cup almond milk or
   dairy milk
1 tbsp vanilla extract
¾ cup almond flour
Pinch of baking powder
Coconut oil or butter for
   frying
2 tbsp fromage frais, crème
   fraîche, or full-fat Greek
   yogurt

Put the cherries in a small saucepan with a splash of water and simmer to make a soft jam. Whisk the eggs, almond milk, and vanilla extract together in a bowl. Then add the almond flour and baking powder and combine well to make a smooth batter.

Place a large nonstick frying pan over medium heat and add a little oil, tipping the pan so that it is evenly coated. When it starts to smoke, add a ladle of the batter, again tipping the pan to spread it over the entire surface. After about a minute, when the underside is golden brown, flip it over and cook the other side for another minute. Serve with the cherries and fromage frais.

Tip: you can use berries instead of cherries or use the berry coulis on page 189.

- **CALORIES** 170
- PROTEIN 6G
- FAT 7G
- FIBER 0G
- CARBS 40G

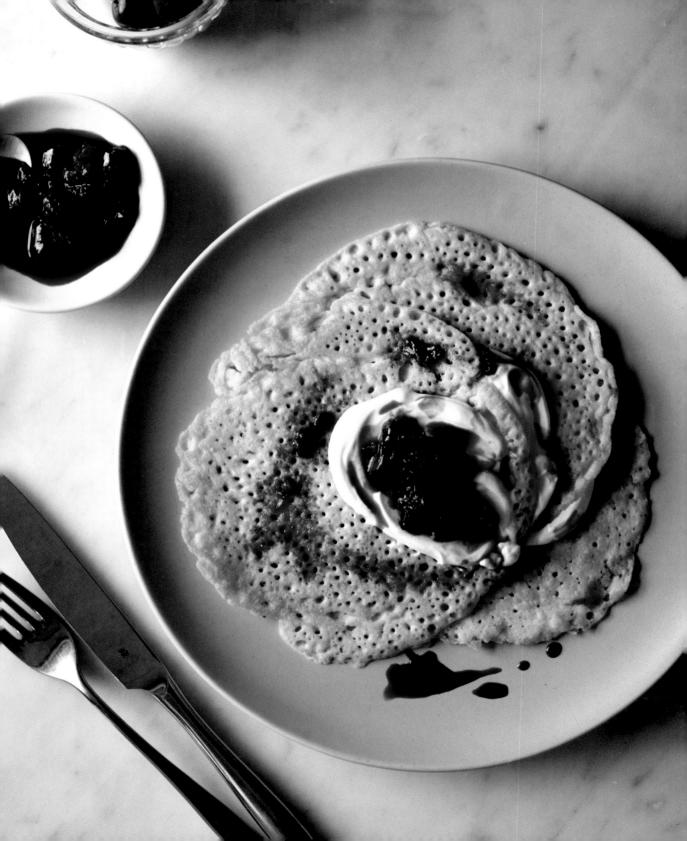

Pumpkin pudding with crunchy nut topping

Inspired by the American classic, this is still full of autumnal flavor, but won't send your blood sugars soaring.

Serves 8

½ small pumpkin (about 1 lb), peeled and diced
4 oz soft dried apricots (about 12), quartered
3 large eggs
¾ cup coconut milk
Juice of half a lemon (and zest, optional)
2 tsp spice mix
2 tbsp pumpkin seeds
2 tbsp pecans, chopped
2 tsp maple syrup (optional)
Pinch of salt

Preheat the oven to 350°F. Place the pumpkin in a baking pan, add a splash of water, and cover the pan with foil. Make a small steam hole in the middle of the foil and bake the pumpkin for 45 minutes. Put it aside to cool. Meanwhile, soak the apricots in hot water for 5 to 10 minutes.

Blend the cooled pumpkin with the apricots, eggs, coconut milk, lemon juice, lemon zest, if using, and spice mix in a food processor. Pour the mixture into 8 ramekins and place them in a shallow baking pan. Pour boiling water into the pan until it comes halfway up the side of the ramekins. Bake them for 30 minutes, then carefully remove the pan from the oven and place the ramekins in the fridge for 3 to 4 hours to completely chill.

Put the pumpkin seeds and pecans in a small ovenproof dish and toss them in the maple syrup, if using. Roast them in the oven for about 15 minutes, or until they turn golden brown. Scatter them on top of the puddings before serving.

Tips: this pudding can also be made with butternut squash, which is available all year round, but try and make the most of pumpkin when it's in season. Baking is better than boiling as it caramelizes the pumpkin/ squash and makes it taste sweeter. For convenience you can now buy bags of ready-diced butternut squash.

- **CALORIES** 140
- PROTEIN 4G
- FAT 10G
- FIBER 2G
- CARBS 8G

Berry coulis or "jam"

A peculiar property of chia is its ability to expand and absorb fluid, forming a clear gel. As it has no particular taste, it takes on the flavors of the other ingredients. So here we use it to make a berry coulis, as a delicious alternative to jam to drizzle into yogurt or over a dessert. It's quick to make and requires no cornstarch for thickening.

Serves 4

*4 oz berries with seeds
(frozen is fine)
1 tsp chia seeds for a
coulis, 2 tsp for "jam"
¼ cup water
½-1 tsp maple syrup
(optional)*

Put the berries and water in a small pan and bring to a boil. When the berries begin to soften, mash them with a fork or potato masher, then add the chia seeds. Simmer the mixture for about 5 minutes, adding more water if it gets too thick. You can add maple syrup for a touch of sweetness if you feel you need to. The coulis/jam can be stored in a jar in the fridge for a few days.

Tip: make a berry "mousse" by stirring half of one serving of berry coulis into 2 tbsp crème fraîche, then drizzling the other half on top. Easy.

- CALORIES 20
- PROTEIN 1G
- FAT 1G
- FIBER 1G
- CARBS 3G

Chocolate kidney bean cake

We cooked this for a bunch of teenagers who liked it and never got close to guessing that the main ingredient was kidney beans.

Serves 12

*1 (14-oz) can red kidney
beans, rinsed and drained
1 tbsp vanilla extract
5 eggs
½ cup plus 2 tbsp coconut
oil
15 soft pitted dates, diced
¼ cup cocoa powder
½ tsp baking soda
1 tsp baking powder
½ tsp ground cinnamon
Pinch of salt
5 oz fresh raspberries or
pitted cherries*

Preheat the oven to 300°F. Grease an 8-inch round cake pan and line the base with lightly greased parchment paper. In a medium bowl, blend the kidney beans, vanilla, 2 eggs, 1 tbsp of water, and the oil until smooth, 4 to 5 minutes. Then add the rest of the ingredients and mix well.

Pour the mixture into the cake pan, gently press the raspberries into the surface, then bake for about 30 minutes. Remove the cake from the oven and let it cool for 10 minutes before turning it out on a rack.

Tip: you can also use this mixture to make cupcakes. Use a 12-cup muffin pan, lined with paper cases. They need slightly less cooking time: 15 to 20 mins.

- CALORIES 250
- PROTEIN 7G
- FAT 16G
- FIBER 4G
- CARBS 20G

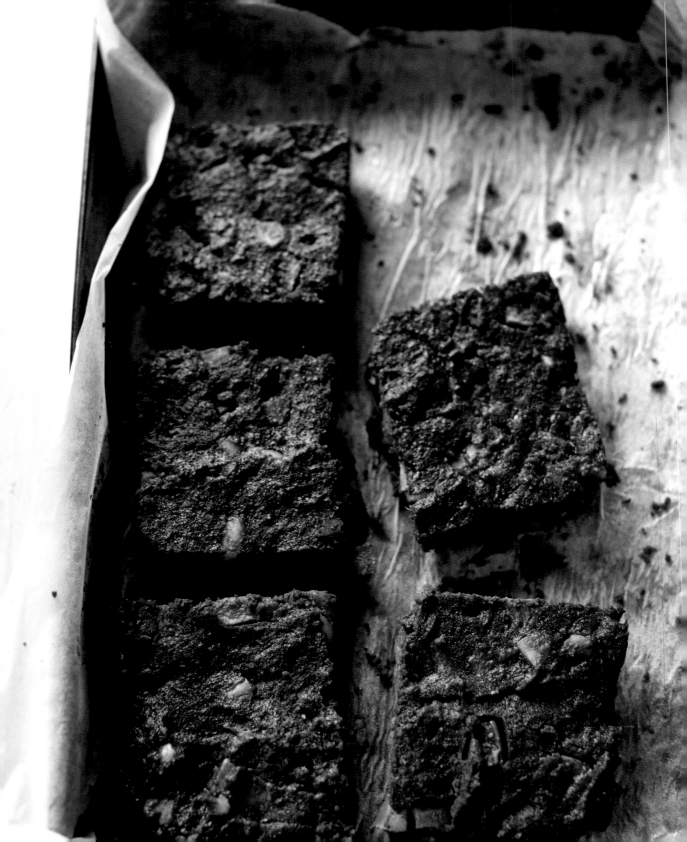

Pear and Brazil nut chocolate brownies

The pear and Brazil nuts give these brownies a lovely subtle flavor. And what's more, Brazil nuts are an excellent source of minerals, particularly selenium (important for thyroid function and the immune system). Cut the brownies small and freeze any leftovers. They make a great after-dinner treat.

Makes 16
(calories are per brownie)

2 oz pitted dates, finely chopped
¼ cup coconut oil (or unsalted butter, softened), plus extra to grease
3 eggs
½ cup ground almonds
1 pear, quartered and cored, skin on
5 oz dark chocolate (70% cocoa solids)
1 oz Brazil nuts, chopped
Pinch of salt

Preheat the oven to 350°F and grease an 8-inch square baking pan. Put the dates in a small saucepan with a splash of water. Cover and simmer for 3 to 5 minutes, or until they soften. Allow them to cool, then blend them with the oil in a food processor or blender. Transfer the mixture to a large bowl and add the eggs, then the almonds, and beat until everything is incorporated. Dice the pear into small pieces and stir it into the mixture.

Melt the dark chocolate in a heatproof bowl set over, but not touching, a pan of steaming water (or microwave it on medium heat for 1 to 2 minutes). Allow it to cool a bit before stirring it into the brownie mixture. Pour the mixture into the pan and bake for 15 to 20 minutes, or until a knife comes out clean. Delicious with a dollop of crème fraîche (adds 90 calories).

- **CALORIES** 155
- PROTEIN 3G
- FAT 12G
- FIBER 1G
- CARBS 10G

A word on fruit and sugar…

For some reason fruit always comes first in the "eat more fruit and vegetables" recommendations. In our view, this is the wrong way round. Unfortunately, some people are eating huge amounts of fruit, believing that it's doing them good. I have seen patients whose blood sugars return to normal simply by cutting right down on their fruit consumption.

Fruit contains lots of beneficial nutrients, but you can almost certainly get these from eating just 1 to 2 portions a day. Try and stick to the lower-sugar fruits, such as berries, grapes, and pears. When you are looking to add flavor or sweetness to a dish, we recommend you go for fruits such as cranberries, prunes, dates, pomegranates, goji berries, raisins, and occasionally, if there is no alternative, a teaspoon of maple syrup or honey.

As you reduce your sugar intake, you will find you start to enjoy different flavors in your food and that you can reduce the tart or bitter taste of some fruit by adding dairy products or the soy or coconut equivalents, which act as a natural sweetener.

We would suggest that you avoid artificial sweeteners entirely. One of the main problems with them is that they are so many times sweeter than normal sugar that they maintain sugar cravings. Ideally, also avoid syrups such as agave or concentrated fruit juice, as these tend to have a very high GI.

When in doubt, go for the whole unprocessed fruit, which is released far more slowly and contains more fiber so has less impact on blood sugars, especially if eaten as part of a meal.

Lychee and pink grapefruit salad

A light exotic-tasting fruit salad which can be assembled in just a few minutes from items you can pull out of the cupboard. Some research suggests that grapefruit helps lower cholesterol.*

Serves 4

1 ¾ cups canned grapefruit in fruit juice, not syrup (pink grapefruit works best)
1 (14-oz) can lychees, drained
Seeds from 2 cardamom pods
½-1 tsp lime zest, ideally in fine strips

Put the grapefruit and its juice in a bowl along with the lychees and the cardamom seeds. To make the lime strips, dig the top edge of a potato peeler into the surface of the lime at an angle and scrape off a fine thread or twist of zest. It looks lovely strewn among the fruit. Alternatively, use a smaller quantity of finely grated zest. If time allows, cover the fruit and leave the flavors to merge for about 30 minutes.

Tip: canned lychees are not always available in the supermarket so grab a few cans when you see them (fresh are delicious if you can find them).

- **CALORIES** 100
- PROTEIN 1G
- FAT 0G
- FIBER 1G
- CARBS 25G

Fruit sponge cake

We cook this at home a lot as it can be made with frozen fruit such as plums, rhubarb, and blackberries. The sponge is made with ground almonds which is the least processed of the almond flours and retains more of its healthy oils and fiber. It has a delicious flavor and a slightly chewy texture, which works well with the baked fruit.

Serves 6

14 oz plums, halved and pitted
½ cup coconut oil or butter
2 eggs
Zest of 1 lemon
4 oz pitted dates, finely chopped
½ cup ground almonds
1 tsp ground cinnamon (optional)
1 tsp baking powder

Preheat the oven to 300°F. Place the fruit in a greased 8-inch ovenproof dish. Beat together the oil, eggs, and lemon zest. Stir in the dates, almonds, cinnamon, if using, and baking powder and mix well. Spoon the mixture on top of the fruit. Bake for 35 to 40 minutes. Serve with 1 tbsp full-fat Greek yogurt (adds 30 calories) or crème fraîche (adds 90 calories).

Tips: frozen fruit is just as healthy and can be more convenient if it is ready chopped. Cinnamon is thought to help reduce blood sugars.

- **CALORIES** 350
- PROTEIN 7G
- FAT 28G
- FIBER 3G
- CARBS 18G

* However, it can interact with certain medications. Please consult your doctor if you are at risk.

Roasted fruit

Roasted peaches (or apricots)

Serves 4

*1 tbsp coconut oil or
butter, plus extra for
greasing
Handful of pistachios,
coarsely crushed or
chopped
4 pitted dates, finely
chopped
4 ripe peaches, or 6 ripe
apricots, halved and
pitted*

Preheat the oven to 350°F. Grease a baking dish with coconut oil. Mix the oil, pistachios, and dates in a bowl. Place the fruit halves in the baking dish cut side up and fill the cavities with the date and nut mixture. Pour ½ cup of water around the fruit and bake for 20 to 30 minutes, or until it starts to brown. Serve with 1 tbsp crème fraîche (adds 90 calories) or Greek yogurt (adds 30 calories).

- **CALORIES** 90
- PROTEIN 2G
- FAT 6G
- FIBER 2G
- CARBS 9G

Roasted rhubarb with ginger

This is so good you might be tempted to lick the dish. The rhubarb and ginger caramelize and char slightly, and are perfect served with a dollop of crème fraîche.

Serves 2

*7 oz rhubarb, cut at an
angle into 1½-inch pieces
1 tbsp coconut oil, or
butter, melted
Piece of ginger in syrup,
drained*

Preheat the oven to 350°F. Spread the rhubarb in a baking pan and pour the oil over it. Slice the ginger into fine matchsticks and scatter them over the rhubarb. Bake the rhubarb for 20 to 30 minutes and serve with 1 tbsp crème fraîche (adds 90 calories) or Greek yogurt (adds 30 calories).

- **CALORIES** 50
- PROTEIN 2G
- FAT 4G
- FIBER 2G
- CARBS 5G

Baked spiced apple with nuts

Serves 2

2 medium firm cooking
  apples
4 Medjool dates, pitted and
  chopped
1 tbsp ground almonds
1 tsp ground cinnamon
½ tsp freshly ground
  nutmeg (if you have it)
½ oz pecans or walnuts,
  chopped
1 tsp vanilla extract

Preheat the oven to 300°F. Core the apples, making the hole about ¾ inch in diameter, so there is enough room for the stuffing, and put them in a baking dish. Place the dates in a small saucepan with 1 tbsp of water and simmer them to form a purée. Stir in the rest of the ingredients, then fill the apples with the mixture. Bake the apples, uncovered, for 40 to 50 minutes. If a knife slides through the flesh fairly easily, they are done. Serve with 1 tbsp Greek yogurt (adds 30 calories) or the coconut or soy equivalent.

- **CALORIES** 260
- PROTEIN 4G
- FAT 13G
- FIBER 4G
- CARBS 33G

Swaps and tips

Carb alternatives

Below is a list of our favorite alternatives to pasta, rice, noodles, and potatoes, some of which you will already have encountered in earlier chapters.

Cauliflower mash

Serves 2

½ medium cauliflower, finely chopped
1 leek, finely sliced (optional)
2 tbsp crème fraîche, or 1 tbsp olive oil

Boil or steam the cauliflower vigorously for 8 minutes, along with the leek, if using. Drain it, and mash it in the same pan with the crème fraîche and some salt and freshly ground black pepper.

- **CALORIES** 140
- PROTEIN 5G
- FAT 1G
- FIBER 4G
- CARBS 4G

White bean or chickpea mash

Serves 2

1 (14-oz) can white beans (such as butter beans, cannellini, or chickpeas), rinsed and drained
1 tbsp crème fraiche
2 tbsp olive oil
1 garlic clove, squeezed (optional)
Zest of half a lemon
Salt and pepper to taste

Simmer the beans in 1 to 2 tbsp of water for about 10 minutes to soften them. Add the creme fraîche, oil, garlic, and lemon zest to the pan and cook the mixture on medium heat for a few more minutes, then mash it well, and season to taste.

- **CALORIES** 290
- PROTEIN 11G
- FAT 17G
- FIBER 8G
- CARBS 24G

Celeriac or rutabaga mash

Serves 2

½ medium celeriac (celery root), peeled and chopped
1 leek, finely sliced (optional)
2 tbsp crème fraîche

Boil the celeriac for 10 minutes. Drain it, mash it in the same pan with the crème fraîche, and season with salt and freshly ground black pepper.

- **CALORIES** 110
- PROTEIN 2G
- FAT 10G
- FIBER 4G
- CARBS 3G

Green lentils

You can use lentils from a can for convenience, but cooked from scratch they tend to have better texture and flavor.

Serves 2

½ small onion, diced
1 tbsp olive oil
3 oz dried green lentils
1 garlic clove, diced (optional)
½ tbsp balsamic vinegar (optional)
¾-1 cup chicken or vegetable stock

Gently fry the onion for a few minutes in the oil, then add the lentils and the garlic, if using, and simmer for 2 minutes more, stirring frequently. Add the vinegar and stock (to cover the lentils by about ½ inch) and simmer for 15 minutes with the lid on. Add a dash of extra water if they are getting dry. Turn off the heat and leave them to steam for another 10 minutes with the lid on. (Or, if there is still plenty of fluid, continue to simmer with the lid off for 5 minutes or so until it has reduced.)

- **CALORIES** 170
- PROTEIN 10G
- FAT 6G
- FIBER 4G
- CARBS 21G

Cauliflower rice
(see page 98)

Zucchini noodles
(See guilt-free spaghetti, page 107)

Quinoa
(see page 99)

Resistant brown rice
(see page 98)

Konjac noodles

Konjac noodles are made from yam and contain remarkably few calories. There are lots of varieties available on the internet or in large supermarkets (though they are more expensive than usual noodles). They come cooked in a package and are best rinsed before use. They have a slightly rubbery texture but no particular flavor of their own so they work best when mixed with strong flavors such as in stir-fries, Asian salads, or soups.

Cabbage "noodles"

This can be used as a base for a stir-fry instead of noodles or rice or with a pasta sauce.

Serves 2

½ small cabbage, halved lengthwise, cored and leaves very finely sliced
Dash of olive oil

Steam, boil, or microwave the cabbage, so that it is tender but still slightly crunchy. Toss it in the oil and season it with freshly ground black pepper.

- **CALORIES** 70
- PROTEIN 3G
- FAT 4G
- FIBER 5G
- CARBS 8G

Tips for when you are eating out

- Dump the burger bun, even if it involves scraping the relish back onto the burger.
- Ask to swap the fries for another portion of vegetables.
- If you have a salad, ask for the dressing on the side so you can choose how much you add. Many restaurant-made dressings are overly sweet.
- Choose the starter and main course and skip the dessert. If you can't resist, ask for extra spoons so you can share with someone else. You get to enjoy the taste, but don't have too much.
- If you have wine, ask the waiter not to top up your glass until it's empty. Alternate sips with water. Ideally avoid alcohol altogether while you're on the diet as this gives your liver a better chance of helping to reduce blood sugars.
- Avoid ordering battered or deep-fried food. Have extra vegetables and greens instead.

What to drink

If you have grown used to soft drinks, or any other kind of sweetened drink, it can be hard at first to make the switch to water, but I can assure you that your taste buds will adjust and you will soon find sugary drinks far too sweet. You can liven up a pitcher of water by adding fresh mint leaves, some pieces of cucumber, even a sprig of rosemary. Fizzy water is fine, too—people often find it good to sip when they are hungry.

Herbal and flavored teas are an excellent way to keep your fluid levels topped up on 800-calorie fast days and can give you a comforting feeling of fullness. (Some people even drink hot water on its own.) You can make extra herbal tea and store it in the fridge to drink cold later.

Remember, too, that milk is back on the agenda. We encourage you to choose low-fat or whole milk as it contains more protein and healthy fat-soluble vitamins. Recent studies suggest that people who consume dairy products may have a reduced risk of developing diabetes and even gaining weight. However, remember that milk does contain a fair number of calories.

The Blood Sugar Diet way of life

For those of you who have lost weight and got your blood sugars where you want them to be—congratulations. Hurrah! That is a fantastic achievement and it will have changed your future in a very positive way.

However, take care not to slip back into your old way of eating. To keep the weight off, we recommend that you follow the principles of the low-carbohydrate, Mediterranean-style way of eating outlined in this book for good. You may not need to count the calories so strictly but will still need to monitor portion sizes and avoid snacking.

In our experience, most people find this approach very manageable. We often hear the phrase, "This is the first diet that I find I can stick to . . ." And that is the secret of long-term success.

8-Week Meal Planner

Week 1

	Breakfast	Lunch	Dinner	
Mon	Perfect scrambled eggs 210	Smoked fish pate with cucumber 270	Thai red curry with cauliflower rice 300	780
Tue	Yogurt, nuts, and berries 200	Tuna wrap 140	Pork in mustard sauce 290 with broccoli, garlic, and anchovy 90	720
Wed	Roasted tomatoes 30 and a boiled egg 80	Halloumi kebabs 430	Michael's fish cakes 130 with mixed leaf salad and Parmesan 120	790
Thur	Green eggs and ham 260	Hummus with vegetable sticks 210	Baked fish with chorizo 270 with Mediterranean vegetables 130	870
Fri	Yogurt, nuts, and berries 200	Tuna and butter bean salad 410	Bolognese 170 and zucchini noodles 40	820
Sat	Avocado with roasted tomatoes 300	Tzatziki with 2 seeded thin crackers 200	Bulgur wheat risotto 330	830
Sun	Apple and cinnamon oatmeal 260	Michael's easy roast chicken 260	Miso soup with leftover chicken 200. Option here to skip the soup and have fruit sponge dessert after the roast 360	720 or 880

Week 2

	Breakfast	Lunch	Dinner	
Mon	Scrambled eggs with mushrooms 230	Speedy spicy beans 250	Salmon with lemon and dill 370 with broccoli and asparagus salad 60	910
Tue	Yogurt, nuts, and berries 200	Feta wrap 370	Zucchini noodles with bacon and beans 270	840
Wed	Kipper and tomatoes 230	Paprika chicken kebabs 190	Cauliflower cheese 450	870
Thur	Yogurt, nuts, and berries 200	Greek salad 190	Turkey burgers 180 with red coleslaw 120	690
Fri	Big mushrooms with feta 130	Vietnamese pho 120	Spicy spinach and lentils 320 with spicy roasted cauliflower 220	790
Sat	Pecan chia oatmeal with raspberries 230	Rainbow salad 120 or option to skip lunch and have the lychee dessert (100) after the korma	Chicken korma with steamed cauli rice 340	690 or 670
Sun	Full English breakfast 330		Moroccan meatballs 390	720

Week 3

	Breakfast	Lunch	Dinner	
Mon	2 simple egg muffins 260	Roasted red pepper soup 150	Zucchini noodles with pesto, goat cheese, and peas 420	830
Tue	2 hard-boiled eggs 160	Chicory with anchovy mayo 170 and seedy bars 80	Beef stir-fry 250 with green beans, soy sauce, and sesame 120	780
Wed	Oatmeal with nut butter 310	Roasted red pepper soup 150	Shrimp pea salad 300	760
Thur	Big mushrooms with feta 130	Piri piri chicken stick 360	Ham steak with red cabbage 420	910
Fri	Yogurt, nuts, and berries 200	Tuna wrap 140	Cajun bean burgers 300 with peas and edamame Yogurt 230	870
Sat	Feta wrap 370		Skinny cottage pie 310	680
Sun	Sardines on avocado mash 370	Speedy spicy beans 250	Piri piri chicken 360 with watercress 10 or option to skip lunch and add roasted peaches 90	980 or 710

Week 4

	Breakfast	Lunch	Dinner	
Mon	Cheese and asparagus omelet 290	Lemon shrimp kebabs 360	Cajun bean burgers 300 with arugula 10	960
Tue	Kipper and tomatoes 230	Gazpacho 100	Chilied chicken drumsticks 410	740
Wed	Yogurt, nuts, and berries 200	Lentil and feta salad 190	Chinese meatballs 160 with greens, bok choy, and oyster sauce 170	720
Thur	Medium oatmeal 290	Endive with anchovy mayo 170 and seedy bars 80	Beef stir-fry 250	790
Fri	Scrambled eggs with smoked salmon 300	Gazpacho 100	Tuna patties 310 with red coleslaw 120	830
Sat	Chia breakfast bircher 340		Lamb hotpot 380 and seedy bars 80	800
Sun	Egg baked in avocado 230		Coq au vin 510 with cauli mash 140	880

Week 5

	Breakfast	Lunch	Dinner	
Mon	Perfect scrambled eggs 210	Ploughman's on a stick 400	Chili squid 160 with rocket and tomato salad 50	820
Tue	Yogurt, nuts, and berries 200	Tuna wrap 140	Chickpea chili 270 with dollop of creme fraiche 90	700
Wed	Kipper and tomatoes 230	Chicken lime laksa 330	Zucchini noodles puttanesca 160	720
Thur	Green eggs and ham 260	Greek salad 190	Salmon with ginger 210 with green beans, soy sauce, and seasme 120	780
Fri	Yogurt, nuts, and berries 200	Chicken lime laksa 330	Beet and fig salad 210	740
Sat	Apple and cinnamon porridge 260	Seedy bars 80	Spanish chicken with chorizo 540	880
Sun	Avocado with roasted tomatoes 300	Chicory with anchovy mayo 170 or option to skip lunch and have almond pancakes (170) after goulash	Hungarian goulash 350 with kimchi 80	900 or 900

Week 6

	Breakfast	Lunch	Dinner	
Mon	Scrambled eggs with mushrooms 230	Tomato, ham, and lentil soup 440	Seafood zucchini noodles 230	900
Tue	Yogurt, nuts, and berries 200	Chinese tofu kebabs 230	Thai red curry with cauli rice 300	730
Wed	Kipper and tomatoes 230	Celeriac and apple soup 320	Chicken drumsticks with garlic crust 440	990
Thur	Yogurt, nuts, and berries 200	Japanese omelet 270	Pork in mustard sauce 290 with greens 30	790
Fri	Big mushrooms with feta 130	Feta wrap 370	Michael's Thai fish cakes 130 with mixed leaf salad and Parmesan 120	750
Sat	Pecan chia oatmeal with raspberries 230	Smoked fish pate with cucumber 270	Chicken and mushroom pie 250	750
Sun	Full English breakfast 330	Chickpea flatbread 110	Chili con carne 260 with celeriac mash 110	810

Week 7

	Breakfast	Lunch	Dinner	
Mon	2 hard-boiled eggs 160	Roasted red pepper soup 150	Spicy spinach and lentils 320 with roasted cauliflower 130	760
Tue	2 simple egg muffins 260	Tzatziki with vegetable sticks 140	Salmon with lemon and dill 370 with broccoli and asparagus salad 60	830
Wed	Oatmeal with nut butter 310	Roasted red pepper soup 150	Turkey burger 180 with Mediterranean veg 130	770
Thur	Roasted tomatoes 30 with a boiled egg 80	Feta wrap 370	Chicken biriani 390	870
Fri	Yogurt, nuts, and berries 200	Paprika chicken kebabs 190	Zucchini noodles with goat cheese, pesto, and peas 420	810
Sat	Avocado and feta wrap 370	Tzatziki with vegetable sticks 140 or option to skip lunch and have the lychee dessert after the lasagna 100	Eggplant lasagna 200	710 or 670
Sun	Sardines on avocado mash 370	Rainbow salad 120	Lamb tagine 420	910

Week 8

	Breakfast	Lunch	Dinner	
Mon	Cheese and asparagus omelet 290	Hummus with vegetable sticks 210	Cajun bean burgers 300 with mixed leaf salad and Parmesan salad 120	920
Tue	Kipper and tomatoes 230	Vietnamese pho 120	Zucchini noodles with tomato meatballs 390	740
Wed	Yogurt, nuts, and berries 200	Poached eggs with spinach 290	Watercress orange and sardine salad 320	810
Thur	Medium oatmeal 290	Vietnamese pho 120	Indian-spiced shrimps 190 with spicy roast cauliflower 220	820
Fri	Scrambled eggs with smoked salmon 300	Tuna and butter bean salad 410	Miso soup 90	800
Sat	Chia breakfast bircher 340		Chinese duck pancakes 340 with greens beans, soy sauce, and sesame 120	800
Sun	Egg baked in avocado 230	Garlicky eggplant with vegetable sticks 90	No pasta lasagna 500	820

Index

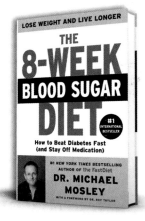